A New Day

A New Day

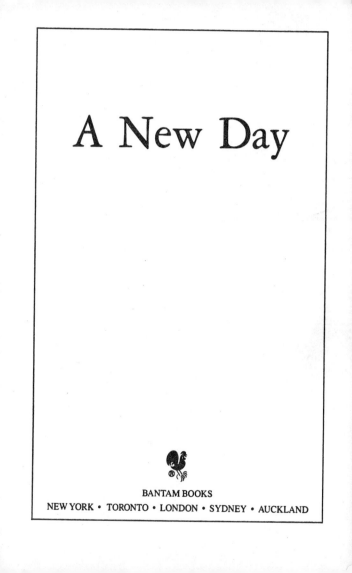

BANTAM BOOKS

NEW YORK • TORONTO • LONDON • SYDNEY • AUCKLAND

A NEW DAY

A Bantam Book / January 1989

Library of Congress Cataloging-in-Publication Data

A new day.

Includes index.
1. Devotional calendars.   I. Title
BV4811.W424   1989   242'.2   88-24195
ISBN 0-553-34591-5 (pbk.)

Published simultaneously in the United States and Canada

Bantam Books are published by Bantam Books, a division of Bantam Doubleday
Dell Publishing Group, Inc. Its trademark, consisting of the words ''Bantam
Books'' and the portrayal of a rooster, is Registered in U.S. Patent and Trade-
mark Office and in other countries. Marca Registrada. Bantam Books, 1540
Broadway, New York, New York 10036.

PRINTED IN THE UNITED STATES OF AMERICA

BM   0   9

Hope is like the sun, which, as we journey toward it, casts the shadow of our burden behind us.

—Samuel Smiles

For a good part of our lives, we were lost, uncomfortable, and blind to the good in the world. There was no middle ground for us. Either we were being funneled into disaster by the tornado of self-will, or we lived in quiet desperation.

All of that has changed. The spiritual way of life has enabled us to be at home and comfortable in the world. Our faith in God has taken the chill from the winds of adversity. We have found the way to peace, no matter what unfolds before us.

In the past, we created conflict and discord wherever we went. We were instigators of unrest, opportunistically taking whatever we could.

Today, because of the kind of people we have become, we are part of life's solutions rather than its problems. We try to give rather than receive, to build up rather than tear down. Whatever situation we enter into, we try to leave it somewhat improved.

The dramatic change within us has become evident to those around us. They are coming to know that our peace of mind and happiness are the result of living a spiritual life.

THOUGHT FOR TODAY: Faith in a Higher Power can be the pathway to peace and happiness.

January 2

When God shuts a door, He opens a window.

—Anonymous

When major unforeseen events occur in our lives, we sometimes have difficulty accepting them. Even though the change may very well improve our lot in life, we're convinced that only dark days lie ahead.

An unexpected job transfer, for example, forces us to move from a coastal location to a city far inland. We dread the thought of making new friends and changing our life-style. Perhaps a treasured relationship ends abruptly, leaving us devastated.

Anyone can be completely thrown by such occurrences, including those of us who pride ourselves on adaptability and acceptance. We turn our eyes upward and ask beseechingly, "Why is this happening?"

Yet somehow, with the help of family, friends, and a loving God, we get through these ordeals a day at a time. Things gradually work out for us and those around us. After a time our lives change in ways we couldn't have planned or even imagined.

When we first faced the changes, we had been deeply upset; it seemed that life would "never be the same." After a while, chances are we've become grateful for the way things have turned out.

THOUGHT FOR TODAY: Nothing is permanent—except change.

A man's first care should be to avoid the reproaches of his own heart.

—Joseph Addison

Sometimes when I think about the past it's almost as though it was all a bad dream. But it wasn't a dream, and it's important for me to remember how harmful my behavior really was. The reproaches I received were well deserved.

Since then my actions and attitudes have changed dramatically for the better. But I've tended to make faster progress with healthy actions than with healthy thinking. My mind still occasionally tries to slip me a Mickey, insisting reproachfully: "You're not doing well enough," "You don't deserve the success you have," "If only they knew what you're really like!"

Fortunately, I've come to realize that I don't have to take those attacks to heart, nor do I have to act on them. When I choose to act, I certainly don't have to punish myself.

As time goes by, my thinking patterns aren't lagging as far behind my behavior patterns as they used to. I'm not having as many self-reproachful thoughts. And when I do, it's easier to tell the difference between a "deserved" reproach for a wrong I've actually committed—and one that's simply an "old tape."

THOUGHT FOR TODAY: Old tapes *can* be erased and re-recorded.

January 4

One's own self is well hidden from one's own self; of all mines of treasure, one's own is the last to be dug up.

—Nietzsche

It was hard to see at the time, but some of us were shaped and propelled through life by outside forces. We assumed roles in response to the behavior of others, and allowed our reactions and responsibilities to consume us. As a result, we missed the opportunity to develop as individuals and to become fulfilled.

We began our spiritual journey with the goal of bettering our lives. But along the way we discovered something unforeseen—our true selves. For the first time we have gotten to know ourselves and have had the chance to *be* ourselves. We have been renewed and in some cases have undergone a rebirth.

Because of our ever-deepening self-awareness, we're now able to shape our lives according to personal needs and objectives. Today we take time to explore and develop capabilities and talents we never knew we had. Consequently, we are able to bring joy, excitement, and wonderment into our own lives as well as the lives of others.

All of this has been possible only because of our willingness to change and our faith and trust in God. As we continue seeking His will for us, we grow and expand as individuals.

THOUGHT FOR TODAY: Self-discovery is one of the most rewarding opportunities of a spiritual life.

Act nothing in a furious passion. It's putting to sea in a storm.

—Thomas Fuller

Once again you've been sucked into the destructive vortex of your own anger. Now the dust is settling and you are nursing a battered psyche, wondering how you can temper your reactions the next time your emotional barometer plummets. Of course, there are no guarantees, but here's a suggested sequence of actions that could make a difference.

First, remove yourself from the situation—physically and, to whatever extent possible, emotionally. This puts you in a position to better understand what is actually happening before you get carried away. Discuss the situation with someone immediately; at the very least, you'll be able to vent your feelings.

Next, ask yourself honestly if you have contributed to the upheaval in any way. Have you somehow provoked or fueled it? If you find that you're even partially responsible, apologize promptly and put it behind you.

If you are angry at someone for something specific, try (as difficult as it may be) to recognize and understand the causes behind his or her hurtful or seemingly irrational actions. The purpose is not to justify the other person's behavior, but rather to see it for what it is. This could help you to react with sympathy rather than anger.

THOUGHT FOR TODAY: There are actions you can take to defuse the self-destructiveness of your own anger.

January 6

Better shun the bait than struggle in the snare.

—John Dryden

When I was still drinking, I always identified with the messages in liquor ads. Even at the end, drinking cheap red wine by the gallon and sleeping on the beach, I was unwilling to let go of the idea of drinking as glamorous, romantic, and sophisticated. That's how strong my denial was.

Even in sobriety, these ads can be seductive. However, when my mind occasionally and briefly veers off the track these days, it doesn't take much thought for me to come back to the reality of my alcoholism.

I was driving along the freeway one day, for example, and saw a huge billboard advertising a brand of tequila. For a second or two, I was captivated by the full shot glass, the exotic and colorful background. As I recall, there were a garland of tropical flowers and a parrot in flight. But most captivating of all was the printed headline: "Anything can happen."

Naturally those words mean something entirely different to me than to normal drinkers. When I read them that day, I almost immediately thought of alcoholic blackouts, of "coming to" in unfamiliar surroundings, of realizing that I was in jail and not knowing *why*.

When I read those words—*anything can happen*—I was reminded that if I pick up a drink, no matter what my motive or rationalization, there's no way of knowing or predicting what will happen to me.

THOUGHT FOR TODAY: When I take the first drink (pill, snort,—*fill in*—), anything can happen.

6

A laugh is worth a hundred groans in any market.

—Charles Lamb

Many of us, as we become honest with ourselves, can begin to see that we take most things in life too seriously. We view our jobs, our "status," our possessions large and small—even life's little mishaps—with far more seriousness than they deserve. The heart of the matter, of course, is that we tend to take ourselves too seriously.

While it's true that many things do require our serious attention, that doesn't mean we have to go about straight-faced and tight-lipped in all areas of our lives. When we are excessively concerned, we limit our ability to have fun, to be relaxed and happy—in short, to enjoy life.

If we find ourselves taking everything too seriously—if we see that we're trying to manage things beyond our control—it's time to reorder our priorities, asking ourselves, "What's really important?"

Perhaps then we can remember that we have a choice: to burden ourselves by viewing everything as "serious" and therefore probably negative—or to strive for a positive outlook, with the goal of enjoying life a day at a time as it unfolds.

THOUGHT FOR TODAY: Lighten up.

January 8

Life appears to me too short to be spent in nursing animosity or registering wrongs.

—Charlotte Brönte

When we first sought spiritual guidance, one of our greatest desires was to "get along." We were sick and tired of fighting everything and everyone; we'd had enough disharmony.

As we've progressed, we've come to realize that true harmony in relationships does not come about simply because we work toward eliminating discord and conflict. Nor does it result solely from "keeping the peace" by passively putting aside differences. Rather, it can be developed through our individual efforts to bring understanding, acceptance, and love to others.

From that standpoint, harmony begins within each of us—it is an inside job. In order to achieve harmonious partnerships, we concentrate on building our own inner resources, instead of expecting and waiting for others to make harmony possible through their actions.

Our greatest strength in this regard, and the underlying foundation of all our progress, is our relationship with God. By relying on Him for direction and wisdom, we are better able to attain harmony within ourselves. Only then can we make loving and harmonious connections with others in our lives.

THOUGHT FOR TODAY: To bring harmony into our relationships with others, we must first achieve harmony within ourselves.

You give but little when you give of your possessions. It is when you give of yourself that you truly give.

—Kahlil Gibran

Yet another blessing of our new lives is being able to freely give of ourselves. We have learned to offer others what has come to mean the most to us—love, empathy, understanding, and kindness.

Needless to say, this knowledge and capability didn't come to us automatically. We first had to take actions to become self-aware and self-honest. For only by truly knowing and understanding ourselves are we able to know and understand others.

We also were taught that the only way to keep what we've received is to give it to others. Initially, we had no idea what that meant. Many of us felt we really had nothing to offer. In some cases, this approached the truth; we hadn't yet learned how to be loving, empathetic, understanding, and kind. Moreover, we had not yet gotten over our early physical and emotional "neediness"—it seemed far more important to receive than to give.

As time has passed and we have grown spiritually, we have found that the opposite is true. Today when we are generous of spirit, we receive far more than we ever have through other means. We feel good about ourselves. We know we are useful and productive. We are close to God.

THOUGHT FOR TODAY: Opportunities to be generous of spirit are always present.

January 10

All rising to great place is by a winding stair.
—Francis Bacon

Every so often we wish we could speed up our recovery. It's been a while now since we've stopped drinking and using, and of course we're grateful to be clean and sober. We only wish we could make equally dramatic progress in the addiction-damaged areas of daily living. We'd like to be less fearful and have more success in our close relationships. It would be wonderful, too, if we could be a lot kinder to ourselves.

We all occasionally want to be—or feel we *should* be—further along than we actually are. Let's remember, though, that just as we didn't reach bottom overnight, we're not going to be able to build a new life all at once.

When we start to get impatient or discouraged, it helps to think back to what we were like in those first days of recovery. Most of us were literally paralyzed with fear and filled with self-hatred. We had no idea how to get along with people or, for that matter, how to live in the real world.

Just as addiction is progressive, so too is recovery. When we compare the way we were with the way we are now, it becomes quickly evident how remarkable our progress actually has been.

No one gets well gracefully. We sometimes stumble or regress temporarily. There are peaks, valleys, and plateaus. But overall, there is movement toward health.

THOUGHT FOR TODAY: If you're impatient with the pace of your recovery, think back to that first day.

Trust your heart . . . Never deny it a hearing. It is the kind of house oracle that often foretells the most important.

—Baltasar Gracián

As I grow closer to God, my intuitive voice becomes stronger. I've learned to pay attention to it, to trust it and act on its urgings. When I avoid a particular situation or person by heeding the warning of my inner voice, for example, I'm invariably glad that I did. Things usually work to my advantage in business matters when I act intuitively. Moreover, following my intuition occasionally will lead me to contact someone who at that very moment is sorely in need of a friend.

In the past my inner voice spoke only infrequently and then usually in a whisper. All too often I ignored its warnings and suggestions. My mind usually drowned out my heart, insisting, "You can handle it—this time it's going to be different."

Because my motives and thoughts these days often parallel my intuition, I am more likely to do what is right and good. I don't end up in places I shouldn't be, doing things I shouldn't be doing. It's so much easier today to make the proper choices. My life has a comfort, flow, and rhythm that I *know* is right.

THOUGHT FOR TODAY: Our hearts often know quickly what our minds find out eventually.

January 12

I believe in the sun—even when it does not shine; I believe in love—even when it is not shown; I believe in God—even when He does not speak.

—Anonymous

Faith has the power to free us of fear and worry. Few things in life stay the same, yet faith can be a constant ally within us.

When stresses and strains pile up and threaten to overwhelm us, we can tap our inherent faith. We can apply faith to overcome negative thinking and to strengthen our contact with God. He in turn provides us with perfect answers and solutions to every question and need.

When we are filled with faith we need not be afraid of any person, situation, or circumstance, for God's power is within us and His grace surrounds us. When we are filled with faith we are positive, confident, and courageous. We can bring our best to all challenges and opportunities as they present themselves. When we tap our inner resources of faith, we are restored, renewed, and refreshed.

Life may not always unfold as we expect; days may not be as bright as we wish. People may disappoint us and we may disappoint ourselves. Yet in all cases, our faith can sustain us. For God is our strength as we move forward in joyful expectation.

THOUGHT FOR TODAY: The power of God is within you, the grace of God surrounds you.

We are so accustomed to wearing a disguise before others that eventually we are unable to recognize ourselves.

—Duc de La Rochefoucauld

Talking with a friend about "people-pleasing," I described the lengths to which I went to gain approval. My friend nodded in recognition. "Yeah, I was that way, too," he said. "For me people-pleasing was people-using."

He went on to tell me about some of the ways he ingratiated himself with others, and the frequency with which he changed his many "disguises."

"Practically every interaction with anybody was motivated to benefit me in some way," he said. "I was always using people. I gave a little—you know, a little kindness, a little attention, even a little generosity—to get back a lot. I played to people's weaknesses and insecurities. It went on like that for years and I didn't even know I was doing it."

Once my friend began turning his life around, taking steps to become honest and self-aware, his old ways of behaving stopped working for him. "It got really uncomfortable," he told me. "I just couldn't live like that anymore.

"These days when I start treating somebody in a certain way and it doesn't feel right," he added, "I have to quickly check my motives. If I find I'm being manipulative—trying to accomplish something for myself—I have to back off."

THOUGHT FOR TODAY: People-pleasing is often people-using.

January 14

A single grateful thought toward heaven is the most complete prayer.

—Gotthold Lessing

Once convinced of the necessity of prayer in our lives, we may be reluctant to begin. Some of us are uncertain and even apprehensive because we've had little or no prior experience with spirituality and prayer. Or we may feel encumbered by our religious upbringing— perhaps by our past disavowal of a particular church or doctrine.

Regardless of our background, one common fear is that if we don't pray "correctly," God won't hear us and our prayers won't work. Some of us are also inhibited by self-consciousness—we feel embarrassed by the whole idea.

When we look to others more experienced, we're reminded and reassured that different people pray in different ways—from elaborate rituals or the repetition of widely known prayers to simply kneeling and expressing thoughts to God.

We eventually discover that prayer is an individual and very personal relationship between each of us and the God of our own understanding—and that it can be as simple as a word or two or as complex as we feel it needs to be.

THOUGHT FOR TODAY: God always listens.

Thou hast not half the power to do me harm, as I have to be hurt.

—William Shakespeare

When someone tries to rile me these days, it's largely up to me whether or not they are successful. In the past I didn't have that choice. Almost invariably, I gave people the power to hurt me.

There was one person in my family, for example, who was forever trying to get a rise out of me. He knew exactly what to say, and he knew exactly how I would react to his taunts. The more upset I became, the more I lost control, and the more power I gave to him. I repeatedly allowed myself to be victimized.

All of that began to change when I became aware that I was being hurt more by my own reaction than by the harmful words or deeds of others. At first I still felt upset when someone pushed my buttons, but my awareness at least enabled me to practice self-restraint.

Over time as my self-esteem rose, I became less vulnerable to unkind remarks or similar negative influences. Moreover, as I became more understanding of others, it grew easier to react compassionately rather than defensively toward the person behind the hurtful act.

THOUGHT FOR TODAY: Lessen the hurt by trying to understand the hurtful person.

January 16

Men who try to do something and fail are infinitely better off than those who try to do nothing and succeed.

—Lloyd James

We all know that risk-taking is necessary to progress. It's hard to disagree with the idea "Nothing ventured, nothing gained." However, it's a lot easier to accept an idea philosophically than to overcome the obstacles that prevent us from trying to do what we want to do.

For a great many people, the most formidable of these obstacles is fear, which in these matters takes various forms. There is ego-generated fear, which tells us that we'd better not take the risk because we might fail—and then we'd "look bad." There is the fear of change and disruption in our lives, which tells us we'll be better off if we don't "rock the boat." And there is self-centered fear, which causes us to worry that we'll lose what we already have, even if we don't particularly want it.

For some, just being able to acknowledge their fear can propel them into action. But many of us have learned that we can approach our new ventures with considerably more self-assurance and strength when we take the further step of relying on God. In these matters as well as all others, we are at our best—and able to succeed most fully—when we seek His infinite wisdom and power.

THOUGHT FOR TODAY: When we don't try something for fear of looking bad, we already look bad to ourselves.

The sound of laughter has always seemed to me the most civilized music in the universe.

—Peter Ustinov

One of our concerns, when we toyed with the idea of giving up drinking, using—whatever the substance—was that life would become serious and boring. We were afraid that we wouldn't have any fun.

Now that we're clean and sober, we realize what it was truly like back then. The images crowd to mind: sitting on a barstool, incommunicado, for six, eight, ten hours. Trying to find drugs at four A.M. Getting it together the next morning in order to get to work. Talk about serious and boring!

Contrary to our fears, life today is rich and exciting. Opportunities abound; where before we spent evenings and weekends wrapped around a bottle, now we're free to enjoy our time.

Of course, we didn't immediately bounce off a solitary barstool into a fun-filled existence. Most of us actually had to learn how to have fun; we had never really experienced it sober. In some cases we had to get out of our own way and stop sabotaging our enjoyment. We had to give ourselves permission to have a good time. Perhaps most challenging, we had to learn how to loosen up and have fun without drugs and alcohol.

THOUGHT FOR TODAY: The starting point for fun is believing you deserve to have it.

January 18

Faith makes the discords of the present the harmonies of the future.

—Robert Collyer

By "letting go" and "letting God," we become free of the burden of trying to accomplish everything ourselves. Rather than relying solely on our own abilities, we take a spiritual approach to our problems and other aspects of our lives.

What are some of the things we actually "let go"? We let go of feelings that cause us pain—frustration, anger, anxiety, and stress, among many others. We let go of preconceived ideas and thoughts that tell us we "can't" receive or accomplish something because we're undeserving or incapable. We let go of old ideas that might prevent us from gaining new awarenesses. We let go of any temptation to resist the changes that are vital to our continuing growth.

When we "let God," positive changes occur. We are relieved of our troubling and painful feelings. We are freed of our limiting ideas and beliefs. Good unfolds before us in the form of new ideas, new ways, and spiritual strength to meet all challenges and opportunities.

When we let go and let God, we do not abandon our responsibilities. To the contrary, we tap into a Divine source of power, inspiration, and wisdom that enables us to more easily meet them.

THOUGHT FOR TODAY: It's not necessary to rely solely on our own limited resources.

Happiness is not having what you want, but wanting what you have.

—Hyman Judah Schactel

All of us know at least several people who desperately seek happiness by constantly attempting to satisfy their insatiable wants. The more they get of the things they want, the more they want and think they need. They move from house to house and from neighborhood to neighborhood. Their cars become more expensive, their jewelry and clothes more stylish, their vacations more exotic.

When we look closely at such people, in most cases it's easy to see that even though they're literally surrounded by all the things anyone could possibly desire, they're utterly miserable. It seems likely that they will remain miserable just as long as they continue believing that happiness can be found in material possessions.

We can feel sorry for them, but we can also feel grateful to have learned one of life's most important lessons: Peace of mind comes not from trying to satisfy our wants as we perceive them, but from accepting life as it unfolds, trusting that a loving God will provide us with what we need.

THOUGHT FOR TODAY: Wants are not necessarily needs.

January 20

Whatever we leave to God, God does and blesses us.
—Henry David Thoreau

As with many concepts, my understanding of gratitude is far different today than it was in the past. As a child I was admonished to think of those less fortunate and to be "grateful" for what I had. Whenever this happened I felt that I had done something wrong, so I grew up with a rather negative perception of gratitude. Even into adulthood I tended to associate gratitude with guilt.

Today gratitude is a very positive force in my life. My understanding of it is a direct outgrowth of my faith and trust in God—a deep appreciation of the blessings He has bestowed upon me.

My most overwhelming feelings of gratitude come during quiet times of spiritual consciousness when I'm able to accept God's grace with humility. Then I recognize my assets and progress in recovery as gifts from Him rather than as the results of my own capabilities.

Naturally, I don't always feel grateful. But I'm aware that if I'm willing to accept things as they are, and to acknowledge my blessings, it's a sure way to feel better—no matter what. In that sense gratitude is a safe harbor to which I can always return.

THOUGHT FOR TODAY: I'm most grateful when I'm closest to God.

Everyone constructs his own bed of nails.

—D. Sutten

It sometimes takes longer than we would like for our negative perceptions of ourselves to change. We should remember, though, that many of us were troubled by low self-esteem for much of our lives. In some instances these feelings were so intense that they caused us to engage constantly in one or another form of self-flagellation.

Now that we're recovering, we're learning to like and even love ourselves. Most of the time, consequently, we're able to avoid self-punishing attitudes and reactions.

However, some of us are so accustomed to our old perceptions of ourselves that we unknowingly hang on to them. We may even take a strange sort of comfort in these familiar old feelings and thoughts. When we do that, we don't have to take risks to find new ways of relating to ourselves.

In my own case, I discovered that feelings of self-loathing begin when my mind feeds me negative ideas about myself. I find that when I can recognize this misinformation for what it is, I don't have to act on it.

Just as I gradually lost self-esteem, so am I gradually developing self-love. It takes time, as all growth processes do, but it steadily gets better.

THOUGHT FOR TODAY: The mind is a wonderful servant, but a terrible master.

January 22

Think for yourselves and let others enjoy the right to do the same.

—Voltaire

Today we want our relationships to be right and healthy. By taking a hard and unflinching look at the ways we interact with others, we've become aware of things we need to work on. One of our most important insights has to do with dependency.

For a dependent relationship to exist, both parties must participate; it's really not possible for one person to become dependent unless the other person acquiesces. We've learned, therefore, to avoid allowing or encouraging others to become overly dependent on us— just as we try not to become overly dependent on others. We have become convinced that the only healthy dependence is dependence on God.

Along with that, we've become increasingly aware that it's not within our power to "fix" another person. So instead of jumping in with a quick answer—or becoming dominant and controlling—we encourage others to make their own decisions and to be responsible for themselves.

When we are able to do that, we give those we care about the right to make mistakes and learn from them—to grow at their own pace. While we gladly offer suggestions and support, we concentrate on steering them toward longer-term spiritual guidance and solutions.

THOUGHT FOR TODAY: In helping others, you're most successful when you show them how to be responsible for themselves.

The true motives of our actions, like the real pipes of an organ, are usually concealed; but the gilded and hollow pretext is pompously placed in the front for show.

—Charles Caleb Colton

Some of us made many unsuccessful attempts to give up drinking, drugs, overeating, and gambling. We tried hard to quit, but always ended up going back to our addictions. A primary reason is that our motives for stopping were misdirected.

We quit drinking because the doctor or judge told us we'd *better* quit. We stopped using drugs because we were afraid our boss or co-workers suspected something. We abstained from overeating to make ourselves more attractive to our spouse. We tried to quit gambling because we were on the verge of losing our family.

All the while we harbored secret reservations about staying stopped. We weren't yet completely willing to do *whatever* was necessary to stay clean, sober, and abstinent. Our real motive was to get off the hook or back in someone's good graces.

All that has changed. We've learned from our own experience, as well as the experience of others, that we can't successfully give up our addictions by trying to do so for somebody else. Today there's no question in our minds that if we expect to have successful recoveries, freedom from dependency has to be our number one priority—*for ourselves.*

THOUGHT FOR TODAY: You forsake lasting recovery if you try to quit for someone else's sake.

January 24

No question is so difficult to answer as that to which the answer is obvious.

—George Bernard Shaw

Some people have difficulty in grasping spiritual concepts, possibly because they try to "find" God by using the familiar tools of logic and intellect—tools better suited for material pursuits. The harder they try, the greater their frustration—and the more remote and incomprehensible God seems. Ultimately, many of these same people come to realize that the first step in finding God is to simply accept His presence on faith alone.

For most of us, acceptance of a loving Higher Power comes more easily with the guidance of others. Since it's hard to believe in something we can't actually see, it is suggested, why not pray to nature, the ocean, giant redwoods, or something else seemingly miraculous?

When we stop trying to understand spiritual concepts as we would scientific theories or traffic laws—when we muster enough faith to at least act "as if"—then we have made an important beginning. Whether we find God or not, we can avail ourselves of His power simply by seeking Him. And soon, by seeing the small miracles that have begun to take place, we can find actual evidence that He is working in our lives.

THOUGHT FOR TODAY: Utilize, don't analyze.

The responsibility of tolerance lies with those who have the wider vision.

—George Eliot

We are all familiar with tolerance as it is generally understood in the legal or constitutional sense. We are aware that it is "necessary" to treat people equally regardless of their color, sex, or creed. We tend to think of tolerance mainly in terms of job equality, equal opportunity, open housing, and so on.

As we progress spiritually the concept of tolerance takes on a new and deeper significance. Our goal today is to go beyond the "democratic" concept to one in which we recognize and respect the opinions and practices of everyone in our lives.

Tolerance at this far more personal level is essential, we believe. If we and those around us are to live comfortably, we must stop fighting and judging everyone and everything. Our goal is to live in the fullest partnership, peace, and fellowship with all men and women. We are all children of God who can form harmonious relationships with each other—if we are willing and honest enough to try.

This may sound like a tall order; obviously, it is not something we can achieve quickly or absolutely. But if we are to further our spiritual growth and remain serene, we must continue striving for true tolerance, one day at a time.

THOUGHT FOR TODAY: The rewards of tolerance at a personal level are serenity, fellowship, and spiritual growth.

January 26

Knowing is not enough; we must apply. Willing is not enough; we must do.

—Goethe

Although I have made considerable progress with many character defects, I still find it difficult to let go of my judgmentalism. It's not that I don't know *how* to let go of it—I've learned from experience that I can become rid of a character defect through my willingness to give it up, followed by a humble request for God to remove it.

When I become self-honest enough to admit that I regularly judge others, I set the stage to ask myself why I haven't yet done something about this hurtful flaw. The answer is that I don't want to give up my judgmentalism because I'm getting something out of it. The truth is that when I judge others, I feel superior to them. And I don't need a Ph.D. in psychology to figure out that if I need to feel superior, I must still have some sense of inferiority.

In any case, if I've gone this far—if I've honestly asked and answered a series of pertinent questions about my judgmentalism—I'm far more likely to do something about it. And I'm also in a better position to take constructive action about my sometimes shaky self-esteem, which clearly remains the underlying problem.

THOUGHT FOR TODAY: Self-honesty sets the stage for willingness and action.

When you resent someone, they live rent-free in your head.
—Unknown

I once had the opportunity to work alongside a man who was going through a painful divorce. Initially I tried to help him forget his troubles by talking about other things, but it quickly became clear that he was so tormented he could think of nothing else.

He repeatedly poured out his bitter resentments: at his ex-wife for the things she was "trying to get," at his ex-wife's attorney for supporting her demands, at his own attorney for not being more responsive to his anguish, at the entire legal system, at himself for having gotten married in the first place.

It was easy to see what was going on. Not just one person, but a whole cast of characters had taken up residence in his head. There was no room for even a brief interlude of serenity, nor for rational thought of any kind. Even if he had been able to rearrange his priorities, it would have been impossible for him to think about reconstructing his life.

Needless to say I learned more about resentment from witnessing that man's suffering than if I had undergone similar experiences myself. When you're filled with resentment, it's usually hard to see what you're doing to yourself. When you see it happening to someone else, it's sometimes a lot easier to get the message.

THOUGHT FOR TODAY: The person you resent probably isn't even aware of it.

January 28

Be still and know that I am God.

—Psalms 46:10

Life is often more complex than we'd like it to be. Sometimes, for example, we start a day with all good intentions, yet everything goes wrong. We look out the window and it's pouring rain. The car won't start. When we finally get to work the boss scolds us for being late and doesn't even want to hear the explanation. Everyone seems to be in a nasty mood.

We grit our teeth and try to get through the day, and of course we eventually do get through it. By then, we have a splitting headache and our stomach is churning. We realize that we've been dealing with situations requiring our best, yet we've been at our anxiety-filled worst.

On days like that, what can we do to change the way we feel? To begin with, we can pause—*really* pause—and sit back, clearing our mind. That may take some time, but it will be worth it. For we can then think realistically about our powerlessness, reminding ourselves that we're not running the show—that it's not even *our* show.

If we can achieve even a small degree of success with those simple actions, we can then ask God to redirect our thinking into paths of calmness. And, no matter what the time, we can start again.

THOUGHT FOR TODAY: A new day can begin anytime.

I have enjoyed the happiness of the world; I have lived and loved.

—Johann Cristoph Friedrich von Schiller

Some people work strenuously and without letup in every area except the one that matters most—*living*. These "workaholics" may be highly successful financially as well as professionally, yet they often end up bankrupt in other areas.

We've all known go-getters who pour every ounce of energy and spirit into their businesses or careers, leaving no time for themselves or their families. We've seen people put their health at risk by literally working themselves to death. Aren't such people missing the whole point of being alive?

When we look at life from a spiritual perspective, it seems clear that our existence was not meant to be one-dimensional. Surely it was not intended that we spend our days with heads bowed and eyes always focused downward. To the contrary, life is designed to be a continuous unfolding of glorious and multidimensional possibilities.

This means that our main order of business should be "to live"—to discover, develop, and enjoy our inner resources. That way we can fully enjoy the rewards of hard work, which go beyond financial security and self-respect. By concentrating on living, we can truly bring "life" into our work.

THOUGHT FOR TODAY: A top priority should be to discover, develop, and enjoy your inner self.

January 30

When you have eliminated the impossible, whatever remains, however improbable, must be the truth.

—Arthur Conan Doyle

When I was young I was led to believe by my parents and others that I didn't measure up, that I hadn't fulfilled my potential— in short, that I never would be quite good enough. Not surprisingly, I grew up with little self-confidence and even less self-esteem. I became an emotional drifter, convinced that I always would be on the outside looking in. My need for approval from others eventually became so great that it was impossible to satisfy, influencing practically all of my thoughts and actions.

After I finally crashed and burned, so to speak, I became willing to listen to others who, to my amazement, had experienced exactly the same feelings. From them I gradually learned to get rid of the "impossibles" in my life: the idea that somehow, someday, I would get approval from those who for so long had withheld it; the idea that any person can be perfect; the idea that I have power over other people's actions or opinions of me.

When I was able to let go of those impossibles (and I still must do so, with God's help, almost daily), I became free to make decisions about my life based on what is good for me, what my real needs are, and what will make me happy. That is to say, the things that are God's will for me.

THOUGHT FOR TODAY: Let go, let God.

To think is easy. To act is difficult. To act as one thinks is the most difficult of all.

—Goethe

There are times when it seems that everything I've learned about the spiritual way of life has flown out the window. Something comes over me and I flatly refuse to practice the principles that have come to mean so much. It's as if I'm a child again, pounding on my high chair while spitting out the food that will nourish me.

I invariably feel like a complete hypocrite following such episodes. On top of that I often compound my temporary regression by beating myself emotionally for not "walking like I talk."

I'm being truly unfair to myself when I react so inflexibly. After all, I am human and can't possibly be willing one hundred percent of the time. I can hardly expect myself to be spiritually "perfect."

It's also important for me to remember that my character defects will probably never disappear entirely. Rather than chastise myself and feel like a hypocrite, I need to think about how far I really have come, and be grateful that my occasional lapses are short-lived.

THOUGHT FOR TODAY: When you feel unwilling, don't punish yourself even more by feeling guilty or hypocritical.

February 1

The little unremembered acts of kindness and love are the best of a good man's life.

—William Wordsworth

We all tend to aspire to and be inspired by enormity and immensity. But no matter where we look we can see that it is the little things that make up the world, hold it together, and provide harmony. The little things also disclose our character and reveal to others what we are like.

Nails, rivets, and spot-welds hold together houses and skyscrapers. Microscopic organisms are the substances of life and eventually of death. In fact, the entire universe—from quasars to the processes of our brains—is in reality invisible electronic impulses.

As we interact in our daily lives, the little things we say and do define us to others and also determine how we feel about ourselves. Small courtesies and simple words sincerely spoken are certainly more effective than grandiosity in reaching out to others. The hint of a smile or slight relaxation of facial muscles can ease a strained situation. A small compliment or the recognition of progress can change the complexion of another's day, and of our own.

THOUGHT FOR TODAY: The true magnitude of life is in the little things we say and do.

The greatest act of faith is when a man decides that he is not God.

—Oliver Wendell Holmes, Jr.

We used to feel that if other people would only listen to us and do things our way, everything would run a lot more smoothly and life would be better for everyone. Of course, it never turned out as we expected. Our past ways of doing things usually resulted in conflict or disaster of one kind or another—even though that's precisely what we hoped to avoid.

Looking back, life was a game to us—a giant baseball game—and we were the omnipotent managers. The problem was that the rest of the team didn't do what we wanted them to, and in fact didn't even recognize our authority.

The players refused to play the positions we assigned them, they struck out when they were supposed to drive in runs, and they ignored everything we tried to teach them. Not surprisingly, season after season we ended up in last place.

Today we firmly believe that any life run on self-will is unlikely to be successful. We have long since stopped trying to play God and have become comfortable in life because we now strive to seek and do *His* will.

THOUGHT FOR TODAY: It's amazing how quickly life improves when we stop trying to be omnipotent.

February 3

Life is partly what we make it, and partly what it is made by the friends whom we choose.

—Tehyi Hseih

I've become willing to listen to others—that's one of the main reasons I've been able to change and grow. These days when friends offer constructive comments or try to steer me in the right direction, I appreciate their attention and concern.

In the past, just the opposite was true. When people expressed concern, I bitterly resented their interference. Rarely would I listen to anyone's advice. On those occasions when listening was unavoidable, I mentally assailed my "critics" rather than even consider their suggestions.

As my downward slide accelerated, those close to me became more and more concerned. Naturally, I felt they were picking on me. Rather than change my attitude and actions, my solution was to change friends. If someone got "on my case," I simply excluded him or her from my life. By associating only with those who would tolerate me, my circle of acquaintances grew ever smaller.

Today I'm grateful for a growing number of true and caring friends. I try to remain open-minded, and have become able to welcome their suggestions just as they welcome mine. I've discovered it's a lot easier to benefit from the experience and knowledge of others than to learn the hard way, by myself.

THOUGHT FOR TODAY: Listening open-mindedly to others is part of being good to yourself.

Prayer is not overcoming God's reluctance; it is laying hold of His highest willingness.

—Richard C. Trench

The concept of a stern and reluctant God is rooted deeply in some of us. Perhaps it has been difficult to let go of the idea that God is judgmental and punishing. We may have felt that God has not forgiven us. Or, because we have not yet forgiven ourselves, we may feel undeserving of His love even now.

Through our own direct experience, we have come to believe that God is loving and caring. It is our firm conviction that He wants us to be happy, joyous, and free.

How do we know this? When we turned to God in a state of surrender and humbly asked for His help, our prayers were answered. We were granted freedom from our pain and obsessions, and were given courage and strength to deal with our gravest problems.

We were led from despair to hope, and shown a way by which our lives and the lives of others could become immeasurably brighter.

Today we absolutely insist on enjoying our relationship with God, for we know with certainty that He is and always will be a positive force in our lives. We pray not to overcome the harsh judgment of a reluctant God, but to join forces with a kind and loving Father.

THOUGHT FOR TODAY: God is all-forgiving, even if you have yet to forgive yourself.

February 5

We are here and it is now: further than that all human knowledge is moonshine.

—H. L. Mencken

Our fears usually have nothing to do with the reality of the present moment—and everything to do with the anticipation of the future. We have to remember that we live and breathe in the present, and need not torment ourselves by negatively anticipating what may occur in the days or years to come.

When we stop and think about it, it's easy to see how negative projection can adversely affect every area of our lives. With a new job, for example, we can become convinced we're going to fail even before we walk through the door on the first day. When we become ill, we expect to get rapidly worse rather than better. As for relationships—well, once again we often expect the worst and, because of our fears, sometimes help the "worst" become reality.

How can we stop ourselves from projecting negatively? First, we can try to come back to the present moment, going so far as saying, "I'm in my kitchen, today is Tuesday . . ." Second, we can recall some of our past projections and realize how we caused ourselves unnecessary pain. Finally, we can remind ourselves that no matter where we go or what we do, God is with us.

THOUGHT FOR TODAY: Negative thoughts about the future bring unnecessary pain into the present.

To live is to be slowly born.

—Antoine de Saint-Exupéry

Our emotions were all over the place in early recovery. We seemed to have almost no control over the intensity and duration of our feelings. They controlled us, rather than the other way around, which is probably why we often acted and reacted inappropriately during the first year. We were likely to be as confused and distraught over a flat tire as over a life-threatening family crisis.

For most of our lives we had been afraid of our feelings, avoiding them whenever and however we could. We had blotted them out with chemicals; we had denied them; we had ignored and sidestepped them. It's no wonder that our emotions were erratic when we experienced them for the first time in sobriety.

It all began to change when we stopped running away from our feelings and became willing to walk through them. With hard work and a lot of help from others, we learned, first, to identify our feelings; second, to understand them; and third, to come to terms with them in constructive rather than destructive ways.

THOUGHT FOR TODAY: When I confront and walk through my erratic emotions is when I begin to regain perspective.

February 7

Never bend your head, always hold it high. Look the world straight in the face.

—Helen Keller

As a teenager I was extremely self-conscious. When I recall those years, I can still feel the emotional pain I endured. One of the most difficult challenges for me was talking face-to-face with other people. I tried hard to sidestep such confrontations, and when they were unavoidable I sought refuge in various mannerisms and techniques that I thought were uniquely mine.

By staring at a person's forehead, ears, or chin, for example, I could escape eye contact. By performing rituals in lighting and smoking cigarettes—or by faked coughing fits—I could lessen the intensity of my fear and discomfort.

One of the most uplifting aspects of my early recovery was discovering that I was hardly unique in my painful self-consciousness. What a relief to be able to laugh along with others who had developed similar techniques to avoid eye contact. And what a bonus to be able to talk about my low self-esteem and fear of people—and to benefit from others' similar stories.

When I stopped trying to hide from people, my self-consciousness gradually diminished. Slowly but surely, my sense of self-worth has risen. Today one of the most valued freedoms I have is being able to easily and fearlessly talk with other people—and to look them squarely in the eye when I do.

THOUGHT FOR TODAY: The best cure for "terminal uniqueness" is to see yourself in another.

It's hard to take yourself too seriously when you look at the world from outer space.
—Thomas K. Mattingly II (*Apollo XVI* astronaut)

Our perspective of life sometimes becomes distorted. It's as if we're viewing the world through the wrong end of a telescope. Compared to the seeming enormity of our plans and designs, everything else appears small and unimportant. We find ourselves taking our problems, possessions, and opinions far too seriously.

When this occasionally happens, it's important for us to take actions that will help put things back into perspective. Of course, we can't all go to outer space, but there are things we can do right where we are to adjust our field of view.

Some of us find it helpful to take a quiet moment—anywhere—to think about the immensity of the universe. We might imagine all the people in the world, in all the households, cities, and countries, and how each person is involved in his or her own life activities. We can envision our life as a continuum—an unbroken span of time. Although each day is significant in and of itself, it is sometimes necessary to see it in context.

When we're able to regain perspective, we find that our experiences are usually more positive—no matter what we're involved in. We have the time and desire to reach out beyond ourselves and to be helpful to others.

THOUGHT FOR TODAY: Take a quiet moment to put your "world" in perspective.

February 9

The most immutable barrier in nature is between one man's thoughts and another's.

—William James

In the past I was almost always in conflict with others, usually because of an inability to deal with my feelings and to communicate them openly. If, for example, I was involved in a disagreement or misunderstanding, I pridefully held my ground and waited for the other person to make the first move. Or if I was on the receiving end of an insensitive remark, I either suppressed my feelings and harbored resentments or immediately went on the attack.

These days I am unwilling to live with unresolved conflicts and the tension they cause. It has become vital for each of us to communicate quickly and forthrightly when misunderstandings occur. As difficult as it often can be, we've learned to put our pride behind us and judiciously say, "Let's talk about it."

By taking the initiative in this way, it becomes possible to better understand others' points of view and to let them know how we feel. We then can work together toward resolving the conflict. In the process we can often accomplish more than simply reducing tension. We can actually deepen and improve our relationships with one another.

THOUGHT FOR TODAY: "Let's talk about it" can resolve conflicts and strengthen relationships.

The fragrance always stays in the hand that gives the rose.
—Hada Bejar

Today I'm going to make a conscious effort to put kindness high on my list of priorities. Throughout the day I'll try to pass along the type of thoughtful and considerate words and actions that I've appreciated receiving myself.

I'll make special efforts to be kind to my family, to my friends, and to the people I work with. When I reach out, it will be with sincerity and interest. My expressions of kindness will be personal, based on what I already know about each person's joys or problems. If I ask questions, I'll be attentive to the answers; as often as possible, my responses will be positive and encouraging.

Instead of being indifferent to strangers, I'll go out of my way to be courteous and friendly. I won't take people for granted, but will try to be understanding and patient.

Starting right now, I'm going to focus on kindness. I'll remember all the ways in which I've been treated kindly—and think about how much those unexpected words and actions have meant to me. Whenever possible, I'll try to make a difference in somebody else's day, and that will make a difference in mine.

THOUGHT FOR TODAY: You will become kind by being kind.

February 11

Making the simple complicated is commonplace; making the complicated simple, awesomely simple, that's creativity.
—Charles Mingus

All too often we find ourselves in a position where we're overwhelmed with responsibilities, concerns, or an impossible work load. There are so many pressing demands on our time and energy that it's difficult to make decisions. Confusion and uncertainty sometimes give way to panic, and we wish we could escape in some way.

Since we can't just walk away, we resort to a more acceptable expression of desperation—we dive in impulsively and try to get everything done at once. Suffice it to say we make almost no progress, while creating even greater havoc for ourselves.

When we're under this kind of pressure, there's a familiar saying that might help turn things around— *First Things First.* By slowing down long enough to apply this principle, we can establish priorities, arrange our time, and introduce order into our day.

Although it's not always easy to put First Things First, when we do we're able to use our time and resources efficiently. It also becomes possible to accomplish far more in a day while eliminating a great deal of stress from our lives.

THOUGHT FOR TODAY: The "First Things First" principle can bring us both a sense of order and serenity.

O Lord, who lends me life, lend me a heart replete with thankfulness.

—William Shakespeare

Sometimes in early recovery we get upset by an unpleasant incident. It may be insignificant, but nevertheless we're bothered.

When our negative feelings begin to mushroom, we feel compelled to get them off our chest. By that time we're almost embarrassed by the whole experience and reluctant to even mention it. When we finally do, our friends tell us several things. First, they too frequently used to get upset over trivial matters, and still do from time to time. Moreover, they caution, a buildup of little upsets is just as likely to push us over the edge as one major adversity.

They tell us that when they get hung up, they take the time to make a "gratitude list," which spells out the positive changes in our lives and reminds us of the ways in which we've been blessed.

Today I'm grateful to be sober.
Today I'm grateful not to be institutionalized.
Today I'm grateful to have been brought back to sanity.
Today I'm grateful for the restored relationship with my family.
Today I'm grateful for my health.
Today I'm grateful to be responsible and self-supporting.
Today I'm grateful to have a place to live.
Today I'm grateful for the way I am learning to feel about myself.
Today I'm grateful for the many friends I have.
Today I'm grateful to have God in my life.

THOUGHT FOR TODAY: When I take the time to make a gratitude list, I invariably feel better.

He that has no real esteem for any of the virtues, can best assume the appearance of them all.

—Charles Caleb Colton

We all know what it feels like when someone tries to manipulate and control us. We're insulted and annoyed when another person resorts to psychological warfare. Of course, it's not always easy to see what's actually taking place when we're the target of mixed messages, subtly disguised dishonesty, or other manipulative tactics. At some point, however, we realize we've been put on the defensive by an intensely egocentric person who is not above deceit to get his or her own way.

Yet as much as we dislike being manipulated, don't we sometimes do the same thing to others? Most people do, although not usually in such calculated and extreme ways. We may, for example, occasionally stretch the truth in the name of expediency. Or we may rationalize our manipulative behavior. We may try to convince others that we're "just trying to be helpful," even though our real motives have to do with self-interest.

It's all too easy to get caught up in the "importance" of our own plans and designs. That's why it's essential to periodically review our actions and examine our motives. Just as we are unwilling to be victimized by someone else's self-seeking actions, we want to avoid becoming manipulative ourselves.

THOUGHT FOR TODAY: If we try to rationalize our manipulative behavior, we manipulate ourselves.

A perfect faith would lift us absolutely above fear.
—George Macdonald

For years I stubbornly insisted that a Power greater than myself could not possibly exist. It was my deeply held conviction that I alone was in charge of my life and destiny. Such was my egocentricity, in fact, that I perceived myself as the center of my universe, responsible for controlling and managing everything in it.

It's no wonder that I was riddled with fear. Although I didn't realize it at the time, I was afraid of almost everything—other people, myself, failure, success, death, life.

Looking back, there was a supreme irony to all of this. On one hand, there I was a blazing star, with all else revolving around me. On the other hand, my fear caused me to feel completely alienated, born out of nothing and going nowhere—drifting aimlessly through the cosmos, yet responsible for my fate.

Providentially, a spiritual awakening eventually opened the door to faith in God. My fear diminished greatly over time as I came to believe that my life was not purposeless, that I was not alone, that I was not solely responsible for my destiny. As my faith has grown, so has my inner security, for I know that God is always with me—guiding, protecting, and caring for me.

THOUGHT FOR TODAY: As my faith increases, my fear decreases.

February 15

True humility is not an abject, groveling, self-despising spirit. It is but a right estimate of ourselves as God sees us.

—Tryon Edwards

Many people have difficulty understanding the concept of humility. Some mistakenly confuse humility with humiliation, for example. They feel that to become humble, one must grovel or be obsequious.

If this isn't so, what then is humility? It is a form of surrender, in the most positive spiritual sense. We gain humility by giving up our pride and self-will in order to seek and do God's will. It is an honest, accurate gauge of our liabilities, weaknesses, strengths, and assets.

One of the most important ways we acquire humility is by accepting our personal limitations. When we are suffering with a character defect or facing adversity, for example, it requires humility on our part to recognize the need to seek help from a Power greater than ourselves.

We find, also, that our willingness to rely on God is strengthened to the degree we can accept our powerlessness in other areas of our lives. Not only are we limited in personal power, but also in our ability to see "the whole picture," as God can. So an important ingredient of humility is our willingness to abandon our own limited objectives and, by placing our trust in God, moving toward His perfect objectives for us.

THOUGHT FOR TODAY: We achieve humility to the degree we surrender our will in order to find—and do—God's will.

My knowledge is like a drop in a vast ocean of promise.

—Tan Sen

Humility is the reverse of pride, in a very real sense. Just as pride is a major character liability, humility heads the list of character assets. Humility breeds such desirable qualities as tolerance, kindness, understanding, patience, and open-mindedness.

Much as we might like to, we can never achieve complete humility—that goes without saying. As with all spiritual objectives, we work toward progress. In the process of gaining more and more humility, however, our lives become enriched in many ways.

In the first place, it becomes immeasurably easier to accept people, places, and things as they actually are. Along with that comes a growing acceptance of ourselves as we are. Because we have a realistic and unalloyed perception of our capabilities and limitations, we become more willing and able to learn from others and to receive guidance from a Higher Power.

Certainly our relationships with other people improve considerably as we acquire greater humility. There is more give-and-take and less friction in our relationships. We see ourselves as equals; consequently we are less apt to be judgmental, demanding, or overly dependent. We get along better not only with others, but with ourselves.

THOUGHT FOR TODAY: Humility unlocks the door to spiritual enrichment.

February 17

If you have knowledge, let others light their candles at it.
—Thomas Fuller

During the first week of my sobriety I was suddenly overcome with an intense desire to drink. I tried to ignore it, but the desire soon turned into an obsession. It seemed inevitable that I would drink; I always had when I felt that way. In desperation I visited the man who had given me support and guidance several shaky days earlier.

"Don't feel bad because you feel like drinking," he said when I arrived. "That's a normal thing for an alcoholic, right? But you don't *have* to drink anymore. That's the point."

My friend then suggested that we "think the drink through." After we mentally took the first one, he asked, "What comes next?"

I couldn't help smiling. "Another drink, of course. And then another. Et cetera."

"Okay," he said. "And where would you end up?"

I thought of some of the things that had happened to me over the years. Suddenly the obsession to drink was gone.

"Where would you end up?" my friend repeated.

"Blackouts," I answered. "Drunk tanks, psych wards, gutters. Standing outside a liquor store at five A.M. waiting for it to open at six. *Sick.*"

It's been many years since my friend suggested that I "think the drink through." These days when I pass the suggestion on to someone else who needs it, it works without fail. And when I occasionally have to use the tool again myself, it's no less effective than it was that first time.

THOUGHT FOR TODAY: One drink is too many; one thousand are not enough.

Self-knowledge is best learned not by contemplation, but by action.

—Goethe

Soon after we begin our recovery, it is suggested that we take an honest and thorough inventory of ourselves. We are urged to put this self-survey of the past and present in writing. That way our behavior patterns and primary character flaws will be clearly revealed, and we'll be able to unload our burden of secrets by sharing them with God and another person.

Many of us are extremely reluctant to take these actions. The last thing we want in early recovery is to be reminded of our past, and to reveal it to someone else. Besides that, we're afraid of what we might find out about ourselves.

When we admit our fears, we're quickly reassured that our past behavior is probably not as bad as we think. Most likely it was no worse than that of our peers, including the person in whom we'll eventually confide.

Then we are told that taking this step is essential if we are to progress in our recovery. We should think of it in those positive and life-enhancing terms, rather than as a negative chore. In addition, other spiritual tools are available to us. They will allow us to progress even further, by freeing us of guilt as well as our actual character defects.

THOUGHT FOR TODAY: Writing a personal inventory is a positive action we take to help ourselves.

February 19

Have patience with all things but first of all with yourself.
—Saint Francis of Sales

When we feel we ought to be more patient with someone, we usually think in terms of restraining ourselves in some way. We tend to equate patience with holding back our annoyance at another person's way of thinking and doing things.

However, patience under any circumstance is not just a matter of self-restraint. It goes much deeper than that. In its fullest sense it is the direct outflow of other positive qualities we have acquired.

When we try to be kind and giving, rather than brittle and uncaring, we are far more likely to be patient. When we have a positive and accepting outlook, rather than an angry "chip-on-the-shoulder" disposition, patience more easily becomes part of our nature. We are apt to have the greatest degree of patience when we try to relate to others with that deepest level of understanding—empathy.

Patience flows more freely when we have faith and trust—not only in the abilities and inner resources of others, but in our own as well. In that regard, becoming more patient with ourselves first requires that we become more kind, understanding, and accepting of ourselves. This is our greatest challenge.

THOUGHT FOR TODAY: Patience is not just self-restraint, but the outflow of kindness, understanding, and acceptance.

Belief in truth begins with doubting all that has hitherto been believed to be true.

—Nietzsche

A woman once lived in an apartment with only one small mirror. The mirror was cracked in such a way that she could see only half of her face. "That was fine with me," she says, "because in those days I thought of myself as half a person."

The woman's low self-esteem soon began to seriously affect all areas of her life. Eventually her unhappiness brought her to her knees and, thankfully, she was able to begin her recovery.

After several months it was suggested that the woman take stock of herself to gauge her progress, to reveal flaws, and to review newfound assets. She was delighted to find that she had changed considerably in a relatively short time. "My fear of people was lessening," she says. "I felt useful for the first time in years."

But she also realized with dismay that she still *perceived* herself as half a person. "I still couldn't bear a full-faced view of myself. Even though all these other changes had occurred, my self-image hadn't kept pace."

She was discouraged, but not for long. Because she had taken the time to be fearless and thorough in her self-examination, she was able to take honest pride in the progress that was so clearly evident. From that point on she concentrated on "getting rid of the small, cracked mirror," and her self-image has steadily improved.

THOUGHT FOR TODAY: Feelings are not facts.

February 21

Whom the Lord loveth, He correcteth.

—Proverbs 3:12

What a relief to know that I'm not solely responsible for "fixing" myself. Through growing faith and experience, I've come to realize that God can do for me what I can't do for myself. This discovery has enabled me to change greatly, and I'm confident I'll be able to make continued progress.

This wasn't always so. In the past I would sincerely try with all my power to change something about myself, but inevitably would fall short. Despite my growing discouragement, again and again I would try to strengthen my commitment and perhaps seek out another self-help approach. The process became totally self-defeating; the harder I tried to effect change, the less confident I became in my ability to do so.

Eventually, I was taught that while *I* can't make changes in myself, faith in God and willingness—rather than more willpower—does make change possible.

These days when I recognize the need for change in my life, I follow guidelines that really work. First, I admit my powerlessness over the situation. Second, I acknowledge my incapability of changing myself. Finally, I ask for God's help and begin to take the necessary action.

THOUGHT FOR TODAY: I cannot; He can; I believe; I'll let Him.

Is it not by love alone that we succeed in penetrating the very essence of a being?

—Igor Stravinsky

Our relationships in the past were sometimes fueled by competitiveness, antagonism, and self-seeking—rather than by sincerity and kindness. Even when we had feelings of love, it was often difficult to express them straightforwardly.

We let our youthful competitiveness spill over into our adult lives—into our careers and even our marriages. In some cases our relationships were based on little more than one-upmanship.

Some of us were able to relate to others only with antagonism. We thrived on keeping friends and family members on the defensive with banter, barbs, and insinuation. Or we tried to establish relationships based solely on what we could get out of them. Our motto was, "It's not what you know but *who* you know."

Our relationships today go far beyond superficialities and negative interplay. Because we allow ourselves to be open and vulnerable, others know it's safe to be that way with us. We are able to establish bonds that are mutually enriching, deep, and lasting. Our approach to others these days is usually motivated by caring and thoughtfulness. We do this not because of some abstract sense of altruism, but because we know in our hearts that these kinds of relationships are the only ones worth having.

THOUGHT FOR TODAY: Nobody wins in relationships based on competitiveness.

February 23

True fortitude I take to be the quiet possession of a man's self, and an undisturbed doing of his duty, whatever evil besets or danger lies in his way.

—John Locke

For most of us, taking the first step by admitting that we had become addicted was extremely difficult. We used every excuse and rationalization, no matter how farfetched, to deny our dependence on alcohol, drugs, food, gambling, or any other substance or behavior. Even after we recognized our denial for what it was, and became willing to change, it wasn't always easy to stay on the road to recovery.

Some of us found our new freedom threatened by the reaction of family members and close friends. In the belief that they were being kind, they said things like, "You weren't *that* bad . . ." "Everyone gets carried away *once* in a while . . ." "You haven't put on *that* much weight."

At first we were tempted to believe them, wondering if what they said might be true. But simply by recalling our last horrible binge, we were quickly able to remind ourselves that we were truly addicted.

We've learned that if we really want to remain free from our addiction, we must be constantly on guard against denial—no matter who serves it up or what form it takes.

THOUGHT FOR TODAY: Denial is a symptom of addiction.

The jealous man poisons his own banquet, and then eats it.
                                        —Duc de La Rochefoucauld

When we become jealous we enter a kind of twisted competition. Regardless of the target of our jealousy, the minute we charge into the arena we have lost. Everything is stacked against us in this one-sided contest, for *we alone* are the adversary.

Our jealousy invariably leads to such corrosive feelings and behavior as anger, obsession, self-pity, and even irrationality. The problem is clearly within us, and has little to do with outside events and influences. Jealousy reflects immaturity, a distorted sense of pride, and, most of all, insecurity.

Some character flaws tend to diminish in a relatively short time. Many of us have found that jealousy is less yielding; becoming free of this self-destructive emotion seems to be a function of long-term personal growth.

We can become less jealous, over time, by practicing spiritual principles. In so doing, we develop humility—a more accurate *perception* of ourselves, and a more accurate *perspective* of ourselves in relation to others. As we build inner security, we are less compelled to react with self-poisoning emotions to outside forces.

THOUGHT FOR TODAY: Jealousy springs more often from our own insecurity than from outside influences.

February 25

*Every beginning is a consequence—every beginning ends
something.*

—Paul Valéry

One of the most pleasing aspects of my new life is how
much easier it has become to accept change. Some
changes are extremely challenging, of course, but at
least I no longer have to agonize through long periods
of confusion and pain before I become willing to let go.

This newfound willingness resulted from being confronted with probably the most difficult choice of my
life: continuing to fail in my desperate attempts to run
the show or deciding to turn my will and life over to
the care of God.

I realized that my old ideas and values were causing
me constant pain, and this awareness caused me to veer
toward the spiritual pathway. But then one night I
heard someone say, "You don't have to change much,
just your entire life."

The prospect of such an enormous undertaking was
so frightening that I almost bolted. It became quickly
apparent, however, that it would be far *more* frightening to remain doomed to my current life of misery.

What I heard that night turned out to be the truth:
I have had to change my entire life. But I haven't had
to do it all at once, or all alone—just a day at a time,
with God's help.

THOUGHT FOR TODAY: With God's help your life
can change monumentally—but only a day at a time.

Fear not that thy life shall come to an end, but rather fear that it shall never have a beginning.

—J. H. Newman

Sometimes we give our possessions and positions far more importance than they deserve. In fact, we actually become tyrannized by our jobs, personal property, and even our relationships. Isn't that what happens when we get to the point where we feel "life won't be worth living" if we lose what we have?

When we hang on to our things with such tenacity, we're left with little energy to really enjoy them. Worse, it becomes almost impossible to let anything new into our lives because we're using so much energy clinging to what we have. That's a pity, for we then miss out on life's true pleasures. We're unable to enjoy God's wonders, the excitement of new friendships and new experiences, peace of mind.

If we're tired of being held captive by our own limited aspirations, it's never too late to begin again. Best of all, we can keep our possessions and positions. There's no need to give up our things, to move to a new place, or to quit our jobs, because real change comes from within.

To begin again and achieve a new freedom, only one thing is required—a willingness to change our attitude concerning what is really important in our lives.

THOUGHT FOR TODAY: Real change comes from within.

February 27

A quiet conscience makes one serene.

—Lord Byron

One of the most effective ways to become free of guilt is by making direct amends for our past wrongs. There are certain situations, however, where our amends may further injure someone we've already harmed. Since we don't want to clear our conscience at the expense of others, we should try to exercise good judgment. We should have sound motives as well as a delicate sense of timing.

If we have been unfaithful, for example, the last thing we want to do is blurt out the details to an unsuspecting partner or spouse. A wiser and more considerate course of action would be to acknowledge our past behavior to a friend or spiritual adviser—and to ask God's forgiveness and help in not repeating our harmful actions. While there are times where such behavior must be disclosed, here again we can be discreet and try to avoid injuring a third party.

The main reason we make amends is to clear away the debris of the past, taking full responsibility for our previous behavior so we can live comfortably and serenely today. Making amends is not a form of self-punishment, but an enriching action that can benefit us and others in the days ahead.

THOUGHT FOR TODAY: Don't clear your conscience at someone else's expense.

The better part of valor is discretion.

—William Shakespeare

Each of us occasionally is harmed or causes harm to others because of our impulsive actions or decisions. We may act quickly and reflexively. Or, without looking ahead to possible consequences, we may simply allow ourselves to be reckless.

Imagine, by way of analogy, that you are on the shore of an unfamiliar frozen lake. Do you immediately dash headlong toward the center to see how far and fast you can slide? Or do you first test the ice to see if it's safe? Further, do you think carefully about possible dangers—including the fact that no one else is around? And what if you've already impulsively started across the lake and the ice has begun to crack beneath you? Do you pay attention and head back—or do you keep going?

While it's true there may be times when impulsive actions can pay off, few will disagree that it's usually far wiser to think things through. We take the time to review the possible consequences of our actions and decisions, even in the face of outside pressures such as the impatience of others.

We also try to stay in touch with our intuition, paying special attention when our inner voice says, "No, don't." And when we find that we've already begun to act impulsively, we try to pull back before we get carried away too far.

THOUGHT FOR TODAY: Pay special attention to your inner voice, especially when it urges restraint.

March 1

God never deceives, but man is deceived whenever he puts too much trust in himself.

—Thomas a Kempis

It's very clear to me today that my unswerving belief in self-sufficiency drew me ever closer to the gates of insanity and death. As a sick, egocentric alcoholic, I denied not only my illness and obvious limitations, but also the possibility that anything beyond my own intellect could be useful to me. I was guided by selfishness, self-centeredness, and pride—the "Ism" of my alcoholism.

What happened was that I finally conceded to my innermost being that I was an alcoholic—and couldn't bring about my own recovery, or for that matter manage my own life. I gradually came to believe that only a Power greater than myself could keep me sober and restore me to sanity.

As time passed I learned that God's power could be applied in *all* areas of my life. I have found that when I seek, follow, and trust God's guidance rather than putting too much trust in myself, I am far less likely to be self-deceived—and far more likely to be comfortable, confident, and free from fear.

THOUGHT FOR TODAY: God's power can work in all areas of your life.

Life only demands from you the strength you possess. Only one feat is possible—not to run away.

—Dag Hammarskjöld

We occasionally hear people say, "Sometimes you just have to stand still and hurt." We've never really liked the sound of that. Haven't we already paid our dues as far as pain is concerned?

Actually, what others are trying to tell us is that there are times when it's necessary to accept things the way they are—even if it involves going through an interval of pain. Sometimes we're absolutely powerless over a situation; there's nothing more we can do about it until it changes. The point is that it *will* change, for nothing ever remains the same.

When we're faced with that type of situation, we may be tempted to revert to our past ways of dealing with something that didn't suit us: we tried every way we could to run away from it. It was unimaginable to stand still and let the pain pass.

It's still difficult, if not impossible, to know how anything good will come from the pain we're enduring. But because of our trust in God, it's not necessary for us to know The only thing we need to know is that He is in charge, that He cares for us, and that we are part of His divine plan.

THOUGHT FOR TODAY: If you run away now, you might miss the miracle.

March 3

The strength and the happiness of a man consists in finding out the way in which God is going, and going in that way, too.

—Henry Ward Beecher

When we decided to seek and do God's will, we weren't quite sure how to go about it. We had come to believe, through growing faith, that He would show us the way to happiness and inner freedom. Now we looked forward to discovering His specific intentions for us, so that we could begin the necessary footwork.

One of the first things we learned was that we had to give up a basic misconception about willpower. In the past we had always believed that we alone could change ourselves and solve our problems—and that the way to do it was through sheer force of will. We used our willpower—or rather, misused it—by trying to bulldoze our way through life.

Today when we face difficulties, we turn first to God. It's not that we believe our willpower no longer has value and should be "discarded." To the contrary, we believe that our willpower has enormous positive potential and can enhance our lives if it is properly used. Through prayer and meditation, we are given guidance and direction by God; by aligning our will with God's will, we are able to carry out His intentions for us.

THOUGHT FOR TODAY: Seek the willingness to conform your will to God's will.

It matters not what you are thought to be, but what you are.
—Publilius Syrus

When I once complained to a friend that I was swamped with work, she smiled tolerantly and said, "You mean this week, right?" She then described a ten-year period during which she had burned herself out as an overachiever. My friend constantly took on far too much responsibility at work, burying herself in projects, *and* taking care of her family. On top of that she volunteered for endless social commitments.

One day during a rare moment of relaxation and clarity, she tried to remember the last time she had had the opportunity to simply relax. She was able to picture herself in action, but not in repose; then she became aware of her frenzied efforts to surpass her own achievements as well as those of others.

"I asked myself why," my friend said, "and I soon realized that for years I had been trying to make up for my imagined inferiority." When she was a child, she recalled, her parents had hardly ever offered recognition or praise. She hadn't graduated from high school and therefore felt "stupid," even though she had accomplished in her life what most people would envy.

"I knew on that day what I had to do," she said. "And since then I've been concentrating my energies on making myself acceptable to *me*."

THOUGHT FOR TODAY: When you're constantly overburdened, take the time to honestly ask yourself *why*.

March 5

Even if you're on the right track, you'll get run over if you just sit there.

—Will Rogers

Since I've now made measurable progress in my new life, at least in my own estimation, I occasionally feel I have the right to be a little complacent. There are times, in fact, when I am tempted to just get by for a while—to go through the motions.

For me, however, there's no such thing as standing still. When I stop moving forward, I begin to backslide without even realizing it. Before long, the small "gift" of complacency I've allowed myself turns into bitterness and ingratitude. I begin to think of all the things I want and don't have, and of the circumstances that are "unfair." Soon I become discontented and start wishing my life were different.

Once I've gotten myself into this rut, there's only one way to get out. I have to remind myself, firmly, that the real problem is not with my life, but with my attitude.

In order to start moving forward, I have to become willing again to recognize and appreciate all I have to be grateful for. Moreover, I need to remember that God has given me unlimited resources. What I choose to do with them makes all the difference in the quality of my life.

THOUGHT FOR TODAY: Complacency leads to ingratitude.

Do not depend on one thing or trust to only one resource, however preeminent.

—Baltasar Gracián

When we think of dependency, what usually comes to mind are addictive substances such as alcohol and cocaine, or addictive behavior patterns such as compulsive overeating. But there are other, less obvious kinds of dependency that can be just as destructive.

What about dependency on people, places, and things? Haven't we all met someone whose self-image and actual identity depend on a job title or a particular make of car? And certainly we know how easy it is to become dependent on a partner for emotional security.

If we're inclined to be overly dependent on people or things, it's usually because we feel inadequate or unsure of ourselves. But unfortunately, when we go outside of ourselves for emotional security, what we end up with is only a *false sense* of security that often becomes a form of bondage. And if the relationship ends or if we lose the job title or exotic car, we're left feeling helpless and empty.

It's less likely that we'll fall into such dependency traps if we have a strong identity and healthy self-image. But these qualities don't come automatically. We have to be willing to work for our personal security and confidence—rather than trying to get them the "easy way" from people, places, or things.

THOUGHT FOR TODAY: Dependency comes in many forms.

March 7

You can close your eyes to reality but not to memories.
                                        —Stanislaw J. Lec

We drank and used, for the most part, in order to avoid painful feelings and to get through difficult experiences. Sadly, along the way we blotted out joy as well as pain.

Although we loved our family members and friends, alcohol and drugs prevented us from experiencing and expressing affection, approval, and out-and-out exuberance. We simply weren't "there" mentally and emotionally.

Some of those people have since passed away. Because we didn't allow ourselves to face and walk through pain, the grieving process was postponed. We never had a chance to say good-bye.

Months or years later, after we get sober, much of the past comes back to haunt us. Even though certain events may have occurred years earlier, it's only in recovery that we have a chance to face and come to terms with our true feelings.

These are sensitive and difficult matters, to be sure. Sometimes, it's hard to make a clear connection between a past event and a present emotion. We may feel embarrassed or afraid; we may be tempted to shut the door on the past. However, by taking care of yesterday's unfinished business, we're able to live with true freedom and serenity today.

THOUGHT FOR TODAY: In recovery we have the opportunity to come to terms with the past.

The past is for us, but the sole terms on which it can become ours are its subordination to the present.
—Ralph Waldo Emerson

Now that we're clean and sober, we're ready to come to terms with our true feelings about people and events from our past. We can't go back and relive relationships and experiences that we missed or mishandled. However, there is a great deal that we can do by way of resolution.

We have found that making amends is an essential and invaluable step. And we can do other things as well to bring about increased freedom and serenity. Today we can truly "be there" for our families and friends, participating fully in their joyful experiences and accomplishments. No less important, we can express the love, pride, approval, and other feelings that were postponed because of our drinking and drug use.

We can say thank you to a friend or family member for help in the past. We can let our children know that we're proud of them for things they may have accomplished years earlier. In sobriety, it may be necessary to go through the grieving process for someone we lost during our days of active addiction.

Whatever the case, we're grateful for the chance to finally take care of things we left undone—to live today free of regret and guilt.

THOUGHT FOR TODAY: Today I can resolve what I mishandled yesterday.

March 9

A theme may seem to have been put aside, but it keeps returning—the same thing modulated, somewhat changed in form.

—Muriel Rukeyser

My attitude when I awaken can shape and color my entire day. If I give power to petty concerns and fears, I am bound to struggle through one self-generated crisis after another. But if I spend the first moments of the morning in meditation—assuring myself that God's power is within me, and that God's grace surrounds me at all times in all places—then it is likely that my day will be carefree and bountiful.

It is possible that I will be diverted; unforeseen pressures and events may threaten my serenity. But even then I will have a choice. I can return to the positive realizations I had earlier.

At such times—indeed, at *any* time—it is comforting to reaffirm this most precious truth: I am a child of God, and God's protection is with me wherever I am, wherever I go. As a child of God, I am free to enjoy my life and all the good within it. I am free to be positive, and enthusiastic, unrestrained by apprehension about any individual or situation. I am free to walk the path of protection and peace and to know that my Father is with me always.

THOUGHT FOR TODAY: We are children of God.

Whenever Nature leaves a hole in a person's mind, she generally plasters it over with a thick coat of self-conceit.
—Henry Wadsworth Longfellow

Every once in a while we get involved with someone whose behavior is an endless exercise in grandiosity. In every area and interaction, he goes to great lengths to show that he is superior—more knowledgeable, more successful, and more deserving than just about anybody. Sometimes he uses the device of comparison; sometimes he exaggerates or lies. Most of the time he boasts unabashedly about one or another of his dubious achievements.

We're uncomfortable when we're around such people, mainly because they put us down—subtly or even openly—to make themselves look good. Eventually, however, our annoyance gives way to sympathy, because we know they're completely unaware of what they're doing. We're reminded of the times when our low self-esteem manifested itself in grandiosity and similar disguises.

What did we uncover when we finally peeled away the camouflage? We found feelings of inadequacy, insecurity, and a poor self-image. We wish that somehow we could quickly convey to such people what we have had to gradually learn through experience. For we're truly grateful that we've found more meaningful and lasting ways to feel good about ourselves.

THOUGHT FOR TODAY: True self-esteem must come from within; all else is temporary patchwork.

March 11

With one man, resignation stores up treasures in heaven; with another man it does but store explosives in the heart.
—Francis Herbert Bradley

All through our lives, and especially when we're young, we're taught that winning is what matters most. "Winning isn't everything," sports heroes tell us with a wink. "It's the *only* thing."

We grew up believing that to become winners we must put our noses to the grindstone and our shoulders to the wheel. We learn to try, try, and try again until, like the little locomotive puffing its way up the grade, we've psyched ourselves into that all-important winning frame of mind.

So it is hardly surprising that for most people the very idea of *surrender* is unthinkable. As for surrendering to *win*, that's not only unthinkable, it's impossible. But the paradox of strength in surrender is true; by giving up our old "selves," we become new, stronger individuals.

In cities and nations across the world, more and more of us are learning to think the unthinkable and thereby achieve the impossible. We are surrendering to win and in so doing are allowing God to do for us what we could not and still cannot do for ourselves.

We are being released from the bondage of self. We are being relieved of our obsessions and addictions. We are being guided into new realms of freedom and serenity.

THOUGHT FOR TODAY: Surrender to win.

There's a divinity that shapes our ends, rough hew them how we will.

—William Shakespeare

The spiritual principle of acceptance can be a solution to all of our problems. Before we can put it into practice, though, we must be able to see things as they actually are. We must be able to discern and acknowledge reality, without the blinders of denial or the distortion of emotional involvement.

In many situations, acceptance means conceding that we are powerless—that as things stand there is absolutely nothing we can do. There are also situations where change is possible and desirable. In those cases, acceptance carries with it responsibility; it requires willingness on our part to take whatever action may be necessary.

In no event, however, does acceptance mean submitting to a degrading situation. Just because we accept our powerlessness to change a person, place, or thing does not mean that we have given up hope, or that we lack choices. We can come to terms mentally and emotionally with an untenable situation by placing it in God's hands.

We can also turn to God when acceptance must be followed by action. At those times we can ask for His guidance in deciding what needs to be done, and His strength to help us courageously bring it about.

THOUGHT FOR TODAY: Acceptance sometimes calls for action, sometimes for inaction, but never submission to degradation.

March 13

There are those who never reason on what they should do, but on what they have done; as if Reason had her eyes behind, and could only see backward.

—Henry Fielding

A major challenge for every practicing alcoholic is to come up with fresh excuses, alibis, and rationalizations to cover his or her tracks. Many of us were amazingly creative and imaginative. We had to be; it was a matter of survival.

I will always remember one such seemingly brilliant but utterly desperate ploy on my part. I had been drunk for hours, wandering aimlessly along deserted streets. It was four A.M. and I should have started for home ten hours earlier. But I hadn't even called. What could I tell them this time?

Suddenly I came up with the answer. I tore at my clothes, ripping sleeves and pockets. Then I rolled around in the gutter, soiling and scraping my face. "Help!" I shouted over and over. "I've been mugged!"

When I became sober several years later, one of my fears was that I had lost my ability to be imaginative. For a time I felt lethargic and empty. "What now?" I wondered. Gradually, though, the lethargy vanished and my mind became increasingly clear. For the first time in years I was able to channel my thoughts and ideas into constructive avenues. I stopped dying and began to live.

THOUGHT FOR TODAY: Today you can use your imagination for life-enhancing rather than life-threatening pursuits.

In the mountains of truth you never climb in vain.

—Nietzsche

Just about everyone is instilled with the idea that honesty is a highly desirable trait. Our notions of honesty naturally differ, depending on our age or experience, but generally relate to specific actions. Children usually point to George Washington and the cherry tree. Adults often define honesty in terms of embezzlement or perhaps a political scandal—and may sometimes describe their own actions of returning a lost wallet or correcting a cashier who offered too much change.

Through personal experiences, many of us have found that self-honesty can be just as important as "cash register" honesty.

There are myriad benefits when we're honest with ourselves about how we feel, how we think, and how we act. We're better able to recognize harmful patterns of thinking such as rationalization and denial. We give ourselves the opportunity to deal constructively with our feelings rather than disguising or evading them. If we sincerely and carefully examine our motives before we act, we're more likely to do the right thing.

We find these rewards well worth working for. We're comfortable most of the time; when we're not, it's easier to see the problem and to do something about it. Because we no longer are hiding anything, we rarely feel guilt or remorse. We are free.

THOUGHT FOR TODAY: Self-honesty has many rewards.

March 15

The universe is change; our life is what our thoughts make of it.

—Marcus Aurelius

Of all the fears we have in life, few are greater than the fear of change. Most of us like knowing what to expect from day to day. We're most comfortable with set patterns and routines.

When change occurs, we tend to think immediately of the adverse ways it might affect us. We fear disruption; we fear learning new methods and procedures. Our negative projections build upon themselves to the point where we lose our serenity.

The fact is, of course, that change is a basic of our existence—the sine qua non of the universe. Although we have no control over most changes that take place in our lives, we certainly have a clear choice when it comes to our attitude regarding change.

At first it's difficult for many of us to accept the necessity of ongoing change in our lives. But once we begin gaining acceptance of this unalterable reality, we can become willing to view changes—both large and small—with an open mind to their potential impact. We can eventually learn to develop positive attitudes. The same energies that we once squandered resisting change can then be channeled into positive and creative pathways.

THOUGHT FOR TODAY: We don't have to adjust to changes all at once—only a day at a time.

The steps of faith fall on the seeming void, but find the rock beneath.

—John Greenleaf Whittier

The pilot has turned off the seatbelt sign and a flight attendant is wheeling a cart of drinks toward you. You're nervous and fearful, but those trays of shiny bottles aren't the problem. What you're really afraid of is going back home to spend a week with your family. It's the first time you've done so since you've become clean and sober.

Will walking into that house stir up the painful feelings you've been working so hard to resolve and put behind you? How will your family treat you? Will they be understanding and supportive about your disease and spiritual recovery? Or will they bring up the past and try to make you feel guilty about it? Will you be able to handle it all, or will you be tempted to drink and use?

If you're planning such a trip and are afraid, the most important thing to remember is this: No matter where you go, or what challenges you may face, God will be with you. He will protect and care for you constantly.

You will also have available the spiritual tools and principles that have kept you clean and sober and comfortable until now. So long as you are willing to use them, they will work for you—at all times and in all places and situations.

THOUGHT FOR TODAY: No matter where you go and whom you meet, God will be at your side.

March 17

Grief is the agony of an instant; the indulgence of grief the blunder of a life.

—Benjamin Disraeli

Self-pity is an emotion we all feel we're "entitled to" from time to time. It's normal and relatively harmless to temporarily feel sorry for ourselves under certain circumstances. The result can be more serious, though, when we indulge in this seemingly innocuous emotion for any extended period.

What actually happens when we're awash in self-pity? We look at things with a limited perspective, for at least two reasons. Our emotions and thoughts are distorted by pain, so the problem seems far worse than it is. And we focus our energies on the problem rather than the solution.

When we yield to self-pity, we offer ourselves an excuse to do nothing. We're not able to get past the point of crisis, nor do we have the willingness to take action to help ourselves. We may stand still for a time, but we usually end up sliding backward.

Beyond those results, if we're filled with "grief" for ourselves, we become distanced from God and spiritual thoughts and actions. There is no room in our hearts and minds to be grateful for the blessings in our lives.

THOUGHT FOR TODAY: Willingness is all it takes to move out of the problem and into the solution.

Love consists in this, that two solitudes protect and touch and greet each other.

—Rainer Maria Rilke

Those of us who were loners worked hard at maintaining that image. We considered our aloofness a badge of distinction, if not actual superiority. The unfortunate reality for most of us, however, was that we were loners because we were afraid, felt "less than," or simply lacked social skills. The longer we remained apart from others, the less able we were to interact—and the more lonely we became.

When the pain of isolation forced us to approach others, we were at first capable of taking only tentative steps. We began by making acquaintances, but by reaching out we soon were able to establish genuine friendships.

Gradually we learned to relate to people at deeper and more spiritually satisfying levels. We accomplished this by being open and honest, and by risking vulnerability as we shared our feelings. As we continued to acquire knowledge and understanding of ourselves and our fellows, we were fulfilled and richly rewarded.

In the past some of us had thought of love as a restrictive condition that could rob us of our individuality. Today as we freely give and receive love, each in his own unique way, we find it to be enhancing rather than inhibiting.

THOUGHT FOR TODAY: Love freely given and freely received is spiritually satisfying.

March 19

Some people will never learn anything, for this reason, because they understand everything too soon.

—Alexander Pope

What would happen if we began to think we "knew it all"? Most obviously, we would stop learning, and that in itself would be a pity. It's probable that we would also become egotistical and arrogant, feeling and acting superior to those around us. If we continued to regress, our attitudes and behavior would alienate us from other people and block us off from God. Eventually, we would become the center of our own limited universe.

Clearly it is far better to remain teachable, not only to avoid such a plight, but because the quality of our lives can continually improve. Life has so much to offer, and aren't we more likely to have an ongoing sense of wonder and enthusiasm if we're receptive to new information and ideas?

When we are willing to learn new solutions, we also can deal more effectively with everyday challenges—and thereby increase the potential for positive changes in our lives. By remaining teachable we continue to learn about ourselves and as a result are better able to help others. Perhaps most important, when we are teachable we broaden and deepen the channel between ourselves and God to more abundantly receive His power and grace.

THOUGHT FOR TODAY: Stay teachable.

When one tugs at a single thing in nature, he finds it attached to the rest of the world.

—John Muir

On this first day of spring, we are especially grateful for the renewal taking place in our lives. Even as the earth yields flourishing plant life, so our human consciousness nurtures and brings forth spiritual abundance.

Everywhere we look, God's miracles are unfolding. Bare branches are clothed with vibrant new foliage; dormant plants blossom, splashing brightness on the fading grayness of winter. The season heralds colorful life in infinite variety.

All about us, change is the order of the day. As we witness God's handiwork in our environment, we are reminded of our own awakening and transformation. Truly we have been brought from darkness into light, from sleep to wakefulness, from sorrow to joy.

Even in the face of day-to-day uncertainties, we are reassured by the order and symmetry of the universe. The unvarying cycles of nature—the precise arrival of this season—remind us of God's ability to bring harmony to all things. Through the orderly unfoldment of nature, we are shown once again that we can rely unreservedly on His wisdom and power, now and forever.

THOUGHT FOR TODAY: Welcome new beginnings —they remind us of God's ability to bring about miracles.

March 21

If you are standing upright, do not worry if your shadow is crooked.

—Chinese proverb

Several years into my recovery I became aware that a person I worked with clearly didn't like me. Although he wasn't overtly hostile, his disdain was quite apparent. What was remarkable about the situation, from my standpoint, was that the man's opinion of me didn't in any way influence my opinion of myself—as it surely would have in the past. The experience gave me an unexpected opportunity to see how much I had changed.

When I began my recovery I was my own worst enemy, repeatedly punishing myself for real or imagined wrongs. If someone even seemed to dislike me, I "knew" they were completely justified in feeling as they did.

Over a period of time I followed suggestions that allowed me to understand myself and give up my destructive actions. As my attitudes and behavior improved, so did my perception of myself. I gained self-respect, and ultimately came to believe in my ability to make the right choices. For the first time in my life I developed trust in myself.

Today, as a result, I'm considerably more comfortable in my own skin. And I'm far less vulnerable to outside influences, no matter what form they take.

THOUGHT FOR TODAY: Other people's opinions of me are none of my business.

We are here to add what we can to life, not to get what we want from it.

—William Osler

The most pernicious thing about our self-centeredness was that it was insatiable. Even when our incessant demands had been temporarily met, we were still afraid we wouldn't have enough. We always wanted more, more, more.

There was no rhyme or reason to our wants and needs. We were as compelled to take pencils and paper clips from work as we were to find "enough" love. Yet as strong as these drives were, we often remained unaware of their true nature and the ruinous effect they had on us.

But today we are aware. We've acknowledged our self-centeredness; we've gained the willingness to keep this tyrannical character defect from ruling our lives. We try to concentrate on what we can put into our relationships and activities, rather than what we can take out of them.

When things aren't going smoothly at work or at home—in any relationship, for that matter—we no longer automatically look for someone to blame. Instead, we try to see what actions we can take to alleviate the problem.

It has become part of our nature to want to feel useful and productive. More and more these days we are there to help others. As a result, we are more fulfilled and secure than ever.

THOUGHT FOR TODAY: The bottomless pit is filled by giving, not by taking.

March 23

When we are unable to find tranquility within ourselves it is useless to seek it elsewhere.

—Duc de La Rochefoucauld

A principal goal today is to become more calm and serene. We're told when we begin our new life that this is a worthy goal, but that we can achieve it only if we seek it in an entirely different way than in the past. We're reminded that true and lasting serenity cannot be found in dependent relationships, through the use of drugs and alcohol, by "getting away," or by accumulating "enough" money. Again and again we're taught that serenity must come from within ourselves—that it's truly an inside job.

At first we were baffled by the idea; it seemed far too abstract. But over time we recognized the validity of the concept. We became willing to see people, places, and things in reality—not just as they affected us. We saw that it was necessary to change the way we related to the world—specifically our attitudes and reactions to it. For many of us, this realization was the first step to achieving and maintaining inner peace.

By making these inner-directed changes, we have begun to acquire acceptance. More and more we can accept things as they really are. As a result our ability to remain calm and serene has increased greatly.

THOUGHT FOR TODAY: Achieving calmness and serenity is an inside job.

Envy, if surrounded on all sides by the brightness of another's prosperity, like the scorpion confined within a circle of fire, will sting itself to death.

—Charles Caleb Colton

When we climb aboard the seesaw of envy, we sink straight down while the focus of our discontent rises above us. In the out-of-balance comparison between what we have and what someone else has, we always find ourselves wanting.

Envy invariably leads to self-pity and ingratitude for what is already ours, as well as disharmony in relationships. We can become so preoccupied with our dissatisfaction, that it's all but impossible to enjoy what we have and what we're doing. Our envious feelings can also lead to bitterness, resentment, and even hostility. It's not at all surprising that the word *envy* is derived from the Latin *invidere*, which means "to look at with malice."

If envy is a problem, it can be helpful to remind yourself that you are a unique creation of God, with your own special capabilities, timetable, and destiny. From that standpoint alone, it makes no sense whatever to compare yourself enviously with others.

Beyond that, an honest and grateful look within, at your own God-given assets, can help you become satisfied with what you have and who you are.

THOUGHT FOR TODAY: If I enviously compare myself with others, I am bound to come up short.

March 25

The heart of him who truly loves is a paradise on earth; he has God in himself, for God is love.
                                        —Félicité Robert de Lamennais

When I think during periods of meditation about the incomprehensibility of God, I am sometimes reminded of Dr. Carl Jung's response when he was asked if he believed in God. He said, "I could not say I believe. I know! I have had the experience of being gripped by something that is stronger than myself, something that people call God."

As a former atheist, it was almost impossible for me to begin to believe in God, let alone to know that He is a part of me. Yet it all began to change when I learned to accept the love of others. That initial receptiveness gradually deepened into spiritual faith, as I embraced the idea that the love of others is in reality God's love.

Today I feel closest to God when I am able to be loving to others. My actions and expressions need not be intensely emotional or dramatic. When I respond to another person with kindness, empathy, or an understanding heart—these are the times when I am most aware of God's love for me and within me.

THOUGHT FOR TODAY: As you pour out God's love to others, it will be replenished by Him in even greater measure.

Sorrows remembered sweeten present joy.

—Robert Pollok

Just because we're recovering doesn't mean we don't have problems. The difference today is that we know what to do; we've been given spiritual tools and we've learned how to use them.

Like everybody else, though, we occasionally overreact when something unexpected happens. Maybe somebody dents the door of our brand new car and doesn't leave a note. Perhaps we tear a ligament and won't be able to ski this season. Or maybe our job promotion means working a different shift. Such events are highly upsetting and can cause extreme reactions, there's no denying it, but in recovery we can't afford to go off the deep end.

One way to quickly regain perspective is to think about where we came from. When we were in the grips of compulsion, our problems were far more severe. Some of us lost jobs, families, and homes. We were in poor physical and emotional health and full of fear. It was all we could do to overcome the compulsion that plagued us.

When we remember what it used to be like, it's hard not to smile at today's "high-class" problems. And it's impossible not to be grateful for the miraculous changes that have taken place in our lives.

THOUGHT FOR TODAY: Compared to yesterday's problems, today's problems are high-class ones.

March 27

To understand one's self is the classic form of consolation; to elude one's self is the romantic.

—George Santayana

A friend of mine decided to buy a motor home and take an extended vacation across the United States. He made sure his home on wheels was equipped with every convenience, from a microwave oven to a VCR. My friend spent weeks planning an itinerary and learning everything he could about his various destinations. He was filled with enthusiasm and seemed more excited and optimistic about his life than he had in years.

Apart from a few postcards, I didn't hear from him for six months. When he finally returned from his trip, I was anxious to hear all about it.

When I asked him how it had gone, he hesitated for a long time. "To be honest," he said ruefully, "it wasn't that great." My friend went on to explain that he took the trip with the hope that his life would change for the better if he got away from his job, his community, and usual routines. Ten thousand miles and a considerable amount of money later, he had learned that he couldn't escape or solve his problems by simply "taking a geographic."

"It was an expensive lesson," he admitted, "but I'm glad I learned once and for all that wherever you go, you take yourself with you."

THOUGHT FOR TODAY: "Taking a geographic" won't solve your problems.

There are no victims, only volunteers.

—Anonymous

When we start doing things that are good and right for ourselves, we become aware of many new choices. Perhaps they were there all along, but we simply couldn't act on them.

Today, for example, if a person offers something that is dangerous for us, we can say no. If we are uncomfortable at a party, we can leave. If the boss asks us at the last minute to work overtime when we have concert tickets, we can explain and say we're sorry.

Other choices, though not quite as obvious, may be even more important. In my own case, a major new choice is not having to "play the game." If somebody verbally attacks me or puts me down, I don't have to be defensive. If I find myself in a "dance of death" relationship, I don't have to keep dancing. In short, I no longer need to compromise my dignity, sink to someone else's level, or put up with abuse.

It takes a while to see these less obvious choices, for they relate primarily to the way we feel about ourselves. The better we feel about ourselves, the more such choices will be available—and the more strength and confidence we'll have to make the right ones.

THOUGHT FOR TODAY: You don't have to "play the game."

March 29

Accidents exist only in our heads, in our limited perceptions.
They are the reflection of the limit of our knowledge.
——Franz Kafka

Open-mindedness has allowed us to perceive the world in a wholly new way. We now believe that God has a plan—that everything happens for a purpose. While the plan and purpose are not always readily apparent, our trust in God helps us to accept their reason and rightness. Needless to say, we are far more secure with this broadened perception than when we saw life as a series of unconnected events.

Of course, it is impossible for us as human beings to envision or understand God's plan in its totality—or, for that matter, from day to day. On occasion life's happenings and their sequence can still seem bewildering and even unfair.

At such times we find assurance by reaffirming our trust in God's infinite wisdom. We remind ourselves that He has all power and that His will is for peace, joy, and harmony in our lives. God will sustain and uplift us as He guides us toward fulfilling our purpose.

THOUGHT FOR TODAY: Be open-minded toward God's plan; it exists, even though it may not be evident.

Every man has a rainy corner in his life, from which bad weather besets him.

—Jean Paul Richter

In the past my lack of self-worth affected my every thought and action. I readily accepted negative messages about myself, especially when those transmissions came from my own mind.

As I began to recover, it was relatively easy to see and change the obvious messages of negativity. Those were the ones telling me I was too fat or too thin when I was neither, that I would always be unpopular, that I had no talent and no future.

It was harder to recognize and then try to change the indirect manifestations of low self-esteem. I refused to buy clothes "in order to save money"—but the real reason was my belief that I didn't deserve new clothes. I didn't make new friends because "I didn't have the time"—but the real reason was my conviction that they wouldn't like me. I remained in a self-destructive relationship so as "not to hurt the other person"—but the real reason for my inaction, more than likely, was the deep-down feeling that I deserved unhappiness.

Today, as an important part of my recovery, I share my occasional feelings of unworthiness with as much self-honesty as I can muster. I try to recognize both kinds of negative messages—the indirect as well as the direct—for the falsehoods that they are.

THOUGHT FOR TODAY: Respect the reality, not the lie.

March 31

A humble knowledge of one's self is a surer road to God than a deep searching of the sciences.

—Thomas a Kempis

A friend and I once spent a long evening with a man in early recovery. It became quickly clear that he was extremely intelligent—he had a Ph.D. in molecular biology. So far he had found it impossible to accept the idea that belief in a Higher Power could bring about not only recovery, but a new way of life.

Each time my friend and I made a suggestion, or shared a personal reminiscence, the man countered with a firm rebuttal based on one or another preconception. We saw that because of the importance he and those around him had always attached to his education and position, he had never learned humility. He was therefore unable to concede his personal powerlessness, and scoffed at the idea that God has all power.

The man was in great anguish, and my friend and I wished there was some way we could magically convey to him in one evening what we had learned through experience over a period of time. But we realized that it was really between him and God—and that at some point he would have to become willing to give up his old ideas. Only then, we knew, could he be relieved of the bondage of self and begin to experience the joys awaiting him.

THOUGHT FOR TODAY: Humility is accepting your own limitations.

You pray in your distress and in your need; would that you might pray also in the fullness of your joy and in your days of abundance.

—Kahlil Gibran

"There are no atheists in foxholes." We've all heard that expression and we know exactly what it means. No matter what our spiritual inclination, we tend to pray more fervently when we feel most threatened and helpless. But after things quiet down, our reliance on God diminishes and we go back to "handling" everything ourselves.

These days we no longer shortchange ourselves by "getting in touch" with God only during times of adversity. In order to broaden and deepen the channel between ourselves and Him, we pray often and consistently. We pray for guidance and knowledge of His will for us. We pray for acceptance, and for courage when action is required. We pray for freedom from fear, and for release from self-bondage. Our prayers are answered.

These are days of abundance for us. Our relationship with God has matured greatly, and our lives have been enriched. We frequently have the comforting and reassuring sense that God is near. In our prayers we express our deepening gratitude for His presence in our lives.

THOUGHT FOR TODAY: God's wisdom and strength is an ever-present reservoir that we can always tap into.

April 2

Think of your own faults the first part of the night when you are awake, and of the faults of others the latter part of the night when you are asleep.

—Chinese proverb

When things aren't going quite right in our lives, we sometimes react by placing the blame on someone or something else. As children we did this automatically to avoid punishment. When we point the finger as adults, however, we do so for entirely different reasons. By "throwing blame around," we try to avoid looking honestly at our own shortcomings and to shirk responsibility for our actions.

If we could somehow put this character flaw behind us with absolute perfection, what might come about? Undoubtedly, our lives would change dramatically. We would be open to countless opportunities to see ourselves as we really are. These new awarenesses, in turn, would allow us to welcome positive changes in our attitudes and behavior. Certainly our relationships would improve greatly as well, for they would be based on honesty and straightforwardness rather than blame and manipulation.

It goes without saying that it's impossible to stop throwing blame around once and for all. Yet if we work steadily toward this objective, we're bound to realize spiritual growth and personal freedom.

THOUGHT FOR TODAY: When we try to camouflage our flaws by blaming others, they only get bigger.

A hurtful act is the transference to others of the degradation which we bear in ourselves.

—Simone Weil

It's easy to see now why my family "walked on eggshells" when I seemed to be having a bad day. They knew from painful experience that I tended to lash out at them when things didn't go my way.

I've come to realize that when I treated others unfairly, it was usually because I was filled with self-centered fear—afraid I would lose something I had, or not get something I wanted. That fear, in turn, triggered my outbursts of anger, jealousy, impatience, and intolerance.

Today when I sense volatile emotions rising to the surface, I stop and ask myself what I'm *really* feeling. Nine times out of ten, I've discovered, the underlying emotion is fear. This realization alone is usually enough to defuse a potentially explosive reaction and put me on the path toward a real solution.

When self-centered fear causes my character defects to come alive, do I still allow my soul-sickness to pour out onto those around me, especially my loved ones? Or do I practice self-restraint and ask God to remove my shortcomings?

THOUGHT FOR TODAY: Unload the gun before fear pulls the trigger.

April 4

Yet through all, we know this tangled skein is in the hands of One who sees the end from the beginning; He shall yet unravel all.
—Alexander Smith

We were bankrupt in every area—mentally, physically, financially, emotionally, and spiritually—when we began our recoveries from addiction. Our minds were confused and our bodies were damaged; a fierce emotional war raged on. Whatever spiritual beliefs we once held had long since atrophied. The spark of our inner spirit was barely discernible.

Although we were grateful to be off the treadmill of addiction one day at a time, the challenge of rebuilding our lives was utterly overwhelming.

We thought it would be best to concentrate first on those areas where our problems seemed most urgent— getting out of debt, getting back our families, getting back in shape. To do that, we were admonished, would be comparable to applying a Band-Aid where major surgery was required.

We were advised to focus instead on an area that was the least known and most mysterious to us—our spiritual condition. As we built a foundation of faith and trust in God, we were assured, everything else would fall into place. It seemed at the time that we were being detoured from our primary concerns. Yet today we realize that the spiritual pathway is indeed the most direct route to stability and health in all areas.

THOUGHT FOR TODAY: Concentrate on your relationship with God, and everything else in your life will fall into place.

I find the great thing in this world is not so much where we stand, as in what direction we are moving.

—Goethe

When we begin to lead a spiritual life we soon realize that we've embarked on a journey without end. We find, to our great relief, that we need no longer seek elusive and sometimes nonexistent destinations. The journey itself provides all the peace and fulfillment we could ever wish for.

If we cannot at first move steadily forward, we can at least keep one foot in front of the other. We do this so as not to regress, for regression can be deadly for us. Soon we become grateful for the necessity that makes us move forward, because we are more than compensated for our effort by the countless gifts we receive.

Our new way of life is a great gift unto itself. As each day unfolds and we apply the principles and techniques we have been taught, we receive countless additional gifts. We learn to live physically and emotionally sober lives. We receive hope, joy, and inner freedom. We acquire special friendships and a deep sense of belonging. We share mutual trust, understanding, and love.

Over time our entire approach to life changes. We willingly accept responsibility. We view problems as opportunities. We instinctively reach out to others. We are grateful to God.

THOUGHT FOR TODAY: The joy is in the journey.

April 6

An emotion ceases to be a passion as soon as we form a clear and distinct idea of it.

—Baruch Spinoza

We're always on the lookout for tools to help us live more comfortably. The most effective ones, we've found, are often those that are uncomplicated and easy to apply. One such tried-and-true tool is to put our thoughts and feelings in writing.

There are a lot of advantages to writing things out. For one thing, it helps us to better understand ourselves. When we put our thoughts and feelings on paper, we can sort them out and deal with them in an organized way, rather than trying to handle them as they float about haphazardly.

Writing can be especially useful during trying times. Problems seem to return to normal size and fall into perspective when we write them down. Listing solutions, alternatives, and pros and cons enables us to visualize exactly what we have to work with. This brings us greater assurance and the ability to make informed choices.

When we put our fears and resentments on paper, we set the stage for sharing them with another person. Once our feelings have become crystallized into actual words that we can see, it's much easier to articulate them. Of course, writing is also an important safety valve. It gives us a chance to vent our anger and to get rid of irrational thoughts before they get out of hand.

THOUGHT FOR TODAY: Negative thoughts and feelings are much more easily dissolved once they've been crystallized in writing.

I see the better course and approve it; I follow the worse.

—Ovid

When I surrender to God's will—when I am able to act in the spirit of, "Thy will, not mine, be done"—those are the times when I am most comfortable and successful.

With God's power sustaining me, I need not rely on my own limited resources. Because I have a clearer and more realistic perspective of unfolding challenges, I am more likely to respond appropriately. I am better able to accept and be grateful for whatever comes my way.

Inevitably, however, there are days when my lifelong enemy, self-will, takes control. Then I insist on doing things my way, because once again I have deceived myself into believing I can and should manage my own life. "This is too small for God to handle," I rationalize. Or, "This is too important." Or, "I'm too busy to establish conscious contact with God, and besides, I don't want to burden Him with my troubles."

The results are always the same. I end up feeling uncomfortable, disillusioned, and perhaps regretful for something I've done.

But over time I've progressed, and have learned this much: When the tug-of-war between my willfulness and my desire to do God's will begins, the sooner I surrender, the sooner I win.

THOUGHT FOR TODAY: Today I will set myself free by surrendering to God's will.

April 8

Men become bad and guilty because they speak and act without foreseeing the results of their words and their deeds.
— Franz Kafka

Self-restraint should be an important goal in our new lives. For some of us, though, it's difficult to achieve. We find that self-restraint is a learned behavior. We have to literally train ourselves to step back and think before we act, until such behavior becomes automatic.

What was automatic in the past was our childish *lack* of restraint. Many of us were impulsive and quick-tempered. At the drop of a hat we lashed out and got into furious arguments or even physical confrontations.

We've since learned that when we "fly off the handle," our ability to be tolerant and fair-minded flies out the window. We've learned that when we act hastily and rashly—without thought—we misrepresent our true selves. We've learned that a single unrestrained outburst can ruin our relationship with another person—and can even affect our lives and futures.

When we begin to make progress in this area and practice self-restraint, we find personal rewards that go beyond the actual conquering moment. We have better relationships with others. People have more respect for us, and we have more respect for ourselves. Most of the time we're more comfortable than we ever could have imagined.

THOUGHT FOR TODAY: Life doesn't have to be a demolition derby.

Be sober, be vigilant; because your adversary the devil, as a roaring lion, walketh about, seeking whom he may devour.
—1 Peter 5:8

Alcoholics and addicts are physiologically, mentally, and emotionally different from those not afflicted with our disease. We carry these differences with us into recovery. Only by accepting them and working with them in positive ways are we able to live sober lives.

Events and circumstances that may have no special effects on so-called normal people, for example, can affect us in dramatic ways. Sickness is a primary case in point. When we are not well—be it from the flu or gum surgery—we tend to become highly vulnerable to our old ideas.

It's all too easy for us at those times to slide backward into the bog of self-pity, looking on the dark side of everything and bleating, "Why me?" If sickness from drinking and using was commonplace in the past, we sometimes feel responsible when we are sick today. We may feel guilty and become depressed.

In my own case, whenever I am sick, my defenses against the first drink are substantially weakened. My alcoholic mind invariably tries to convince me that a few drinks would help me to feel better. That's why when I'm ill, I make special efforts to keep sobriety my number one priority.

THOUGHT FOR TODAY: Old ideas are insidious, powerful—and patient.

April 10

*Not all things have to be scrutinized, nor all friends tested,
nor all enemies exposed and denounced.*

—Spanish proverb

We all have a tendency to want others to do things our
way. Without necessarily realizing it, we sometimes
expect people to live by our ideals and standards. When
they don't, we're inclined to be judgmental and critical
of their "shortcomings." Taking that a step further, we
feel it's our right and perhaps even our *duty* to fight
back when we feel we've been offended, directly or
indirectly, by another person's behavior.

But when we do this, aren't we taking on something
beyond our control? Aren't we actually fighting ourselves? When we act on our judgments by trying to
change other people, we're the ones who are injured.
Almost always, we're unsuccessful—and we end up
feeling even greater resentment and self-pity.

The truth is, no person ever changes attitudes or
behavior until he or she has a desire to change. Moreover, in most cases we really don't know another person's background, and thereby can't fully understand
his or her motives or the forces that shaped them. What
right, then, do we have to judge that person?

That's why it's vital to our serenity to allow others to
live their lives while we live ours—to *live and let live*.

THOUGHT FOR TODAY: Fighting another person's
"shortcomings" is like shadowboxing; we're the ones who
sweat and get worn out.

In judging of others a man labors in vain, often errs, and easily sins; but in judging and examining himself, he always labors fruitfully.

—Thomas a Kempis

"Live and let live." What does this familiar slogan actually mean? How can we put it to use in our daily lives?

We can begin by concentrating on the first word—*live*. It tells us to enjoy our lives fully, despite what other people around us are doing or not doing. When we enrich our days with fulfilling activities, we're less inclined to be negatively influenced by outside forces. Furthermore, we are not as likely to criticize and judge others. In short, our priority is getting the most out of life by growing spiritually.

Clearly, though, it's all but impossible to move forward if we continually allow ourselves to be upset or offended by the behavior and attitudes of other people. This brings us to the words *let live*. Here we begin by accepting our powerlessness over others. We acknowledge the right of every person to live as he or she chooses, free from our criticism, judgment, contempt, and resentment.

Needless to say, it's a formidable challenge to totally change our attitude toward those who are upsetting us. It takes time and discipline, to be sure, but the results will most assuredly be rewarding.

THOUGHT FOR TODAY: When we concentrate on our own lives, we're less likely to scrutinize the way others live.

April 12

Formidable is that enemy that lies hid in a man's own heart.
—Publilius Syrus

If anyone had ever treated me as badly as I treated myself, I would have considered him an archenemy. As it turned out, *I* was that enemy. Because of the way I felt about myself, I became enmeshed in my own web of self-hatred, self-destruction, and self-recrimination.

When I was finally able to stop behaving and thinking in ways that exacerbated my self-loathing, those feelings diminished greatly. However, they never have disappeared entirely, and I suspect they never will.

In order to constructively deal with these deeply grooved and recurring feelings of self-hatred, I turn and return often to God as I understand Him. I remind myself that His love for me is abiding, no matter how I feel about myself.

In addition to that, I have learned that on my own I make very slow progress in ridding myself of my negative feelings. But when I ask God to release me from them, He does so time and time again. He accepts me and loves me totally as I am, and He has long since forgiven me for real or imagined wrongs of the past.

THOUGHT FOR TODAY: God's love transcends self-hatred; God's power can help remove it.

In certain moments a single almost insignificant sorrow may, by association, bring together all the little relics of pain and discomfort, bodily and mental, that we have endured even from infancy.

—Samuel Taylor Coleridge

Occasionally we experience something that returns us instantly to the old life and the way it used to be. The experience need not be a jolting one with wailing sirens and flashing red lights, or even a sad one.

A long-forgotten odor, a musical phrase or other sound—perhaps the closing of a door—can cause that sense of déjà vu, transporting us back to the state of desperation from which we truly believed there could be no escape.

When the sensation passes and we return to the present, are we filled with deep and almost overflowing gratitude for the lives we lead today? Do we thank God for reminding us of what it used to be like, and for the way it is now?

Let us pause and savor the moment, reflecting on the blessings we have been given. Let us vow to pass our gifts to others, for we have learned that we cannot keep them unless we give them away.

THOUGHT FOR TODAY: Remember the way it used to be, and be thankful for today.

April 14

Once the game is over, the king and the pawn go back in the same box.

—Italian saying

Unlike virtually any other illness, alcoholism and similar addictions are characterized by denial. From the beginning, the addicted person becomes increasingly convinced that he or she isn't sick at all.

Even in the face of such glaringly obvious consequences as hospitalizations, arrests, and destroyed relationships, practicing alcoholics and addicts refuse to acknowledge that there's a problem. They look to every imaginable excuse, alibi, and rationalization to deny their dependencies.

Rare is the person in recovery who does not soon understand that denial is a primary symptom of the illness. When recovering people look back, they find it hard to believe they came up with such transparent rationalizations as, "It's necessary for my job," "Everybody overdoes it once in a while," "I don't ever drink in the morning," "I'm too young to have a problem," "I can stop anytime I want to."

In my own case, I used all of those excuses—even the ones that were outright lies. But for years my number one rationalization was that I still had a job, a bank account, a family. To me, alcoholics had lost everything and were on the street. I hadn't yet lost anything material, so I couldn't be an alcoholic. Right?

THOUGHT FOR TODAY: Skid row is not only a place; it's also a state of mind.

Look everywhere with your eyes; but with your soul never look at many things, but at one.

—V. V. Rozinov

When I first heard others talk about God, it seemed that each person's concept of a Higher Power was unlike that of every other person's concept. However, when I stopped comparing differences and began listening for similarities, I realized they all perceived God as part of themselves.

The idea had great appeal for me. I immediately wanted what my new friends had, because at the time I was still searching unsuccessfully for God outside of myself. It turned out that I had to continue doing so for some time, until I was able to identify and then discard those things that blocked me from Him.

I came to understand that I was attempting to fill a spiritual void by accumulating material possessions, by acting like a big shot, and by pretending that such character flaws as pride and anger were working in my life.

When I was able to abandon such beliefs and actions, my attitude and outlook on life began to change. Gradually, through personal experience, a new awareness developed: *It is only deep down within us that God can be found.*

THOUGHT FOR TODAY: God is within.

April 16

We never seek things for themselves but for the search.
—Blaise Pascal

We spend much of our lives and waste much of our time trying to be in control. We often feel that because we've taken all the right steps and have the best of intentions, our projects and involvements should turn out exactly as we've planned. We not only expect them to turn out that way, we count on it.

As we all know, that's not the way things usually work. And if we expect them to work that way, we're setting ourselves up for a continuing series of disappointments.

Suppose we've finally decided to repair a badly strained family relationship. We do everything in our power to make things right. But then, instead of stepping back, we're tempted to do just a little bit more—and in some way manipulate and thereby control the outcome of our actions.

Experience has shown that trying to take that extra step is invariably a mistake. We've found that by doing the footwork as well as we can—and then leaving the results up to God—we put ourselves in the best possible position for success.

THOUGHT FOR TODAY: Stay out of the results.

The eyes of other people are the eyes that ruin us. If all but myself were blind, I should want neither fine clothes, fine houses, nor fine furniture.

—Benjamin Franklin

Sometimes I read about a person who is "held in high esteem" by friends and associates. I've always liked the sound of that, but I now realize that the esteem of others isn't anywhere near as important as my own self-esteem.

Some of us learned this the hard way. For years we went to great lengths to become highly thought of. Our decisions in many areas often were motivated solely by that objective. The clothes we wore, the way we talked and acted—even our career choices—were strongly influenced by our need to fit in, to win approval, to make the right impression.

We gave up a lot in order to "look good," frequently ignoring opportunities that would have helped us to develop a sense of self. In some cases we never got to know our true opinions, tastes, and aspirations. We never did get any real satisfactions; what we were after was not only ephemeral but, in the long run, unobtainable.

Today we try to make decisions based on our knowledge of what's right and good. Regardless of outside pressures—the "eyes of others"—we know that the greatest satisfaction in life comes from being true to ourselves.

THOUGHT FOR TODAY: Make the right impression—on yourself.

April 18

Happiness itself is a kind of gratitude.

—Joseph Wood Krutch

For a long time, I believed my personal triumphs were solely the result of my own talents and abilities. If credit was to be given, it had to be given to me. When I achieved even limited successes, nobody applauded longer and more loudly than I.

I took it for granted at a young age that achievements would always come easily to me. At school and early in my career, for example, I did well with very little effort—and consequently was forever patting myself on the back. Ultimately, however, my egocentricity was my undoing. It took a steep downward plunge and considerable suffering before I could admit defeat and become willing to try a new way.

When I began living a spiritual life, I soon learned some important lessons about gratitude. Through the miraculous experience of recovery, I began to understand that all my successes are God-given, as are my talents and abilities.

Today I try to give credit where credit is due. And I find that when I am filled with gratitude for God's blessings, rather than self-adulation, I am more apt to be conscious of His presence.

THOUGHT FOR TODAY: The credit belongs to God.

The misfortunes hardest to bear are those which never come.
—J. R. Lowell

Long after most other fears have diminished or disappeared, the fear of financial insecurity often lingers. Perhaps that's because it takes a while to realize that the problem isn't financial insecurity at all—it's the fear of it.

Those who are wealthy can be just as obsessed about finances as those who are actually strapped for cash. Fear of financial insecurity has nothing to do with economic status, but is like any other form of self-centered fear: We're afraid we will lose something we have, or we're afraid we won't get something we want.

Clearly then, to regain a sense of well-being, we need to concentrate not on our bank balance, but on our phantom fears. The first thing we might do is step back from our emotional involvement with the "problem." That way we can look at things as they really are, instead of letting our imaginations run wild.

Most important, we can turn to God and ask for His help. We know from experience that fear can be effectively overcome and replaced by faith. We also know that God will provide for us, no matter what. If we trust that He will continue to do so, and act in faith by doing what is put in front of us, our fears will leave us.

THOUGHT FOR TODAY: Most of our fears have nothing to do with reality.

April 20

He who can not forgive others breaks the bridge over which he must pass himself.

—George Herbert

The importance of practicing forgiveness has been a spiritual axiom throughout the ages. Prophets, saints, and Scripture admonish us to forgive; the principle is a mainstay of virtually every religious and philosophical doctrine.

Why is it so important to forgive a person who has wronged us? When we offer forgiveness, we are able to constructively deal with our feelings of hurt, resentment, and self-pity—and are less likely to compound these difficulties. But if we hold a grudge against someone, we end up bearing a heavy burden that restricts our freedom and holds us back from spiritual growth.

Few people will argue against the importance and desirability of forgiveness. As with many concepts, however, it is often difficult to put into practice.

We can set the stage for forgiveness by first trying to be understanding of those who have wronged us. To achieve understanding, it is helpful to acknowledge that because we are human and fallible, we're entirely capable of committing a similar wrong. At some future time, therefore, we also may need to be forgiven. If God can forgive those who have wronged us, then we can, too.

THOUGHT FOR TODAY: Forgiveness brings about freedom.

Let me tell you the secret that has led me to my goal. My strength lies solely in my tenacity.

—Louis Pasteur

While some changes in our lives have taken place quickly—even miraculously—others have taken longer and have required considerable effort on our part.

Many of us tried fruitlessly for years to free ourselves of addictions, to alter destructive behavior patterns, or simply to improve our lives. It was not until we became entirely willing to change, and then sought help through God's wisdom and strength, that we experienced positive results.

An absolutely essential ingredient in this process, we discovered, is hard work and discipline on our part. We no longer try to will our problems away, nor do we sit back passively and expect God to do it all. We've learned that action is the necessary catalyst in changing lifelong patterns.

Some of us, for example, have suffered greatly because of our frequent angry outbursts. Today we're making progress, and are far less likely to behave explosively. This is not only because of God's invaluable help, but also because of our disciplined and tenacious efforts to practice self-restraint. Day by day, working in partnership with God, our successes increase.

THOUGHT FOR TODAY: God can certainly help you to change, but not without both willingness and action on your part.

April 22

Trouble and perplexity drive me to prayer, and prayer drives away perplexity and trouble.
                    —Philipp Schwarzert Melanchthon

Sometimes I fall into the habit of giving short shrift to God. Because my life has gotten unusually busy, or for other reasons, I neglect my relationship with Him. I can't seem to find time to meditate. I pray on the run, if at all, perhaps when I'm shaving, or while driving on the freeway with the radio playing.

If this goes on for any length of time, the quality of my life is negatively affected. Little things start to bother me in big ways. I become impatient and short-tempered; my ego starts getting out of hand. My discomfort builds and builds, until I finally realize what the problem is.

At that point I have to get back in shape spiritually. Just as it takes regular exercise for me to stay physically fit, so it takes regular prayer and meditation to stay emotionally and spiritually fit.

Today I will step aside from the mainstream of activity. In a quiet place and with a tranquil mind, I will retreat with God in order to strengthen my inner life.

THOUGHT FOR TODAY: EGO = Edging God Out.

Character is much easier kept than recovered.

—Thomas Paine

Do we sometimes react childishly when things don't go our way? For most of us, if we stop and think about it, the honest answer would probably be "Yes."

Don't we sometimes interrupt people before they are finished talking—because we feel what we have to say is more important? Don't we stubbornly try to bulldog others into coming around to *our* point of view? And aren't we occasionally spoilsports when we come out second- or third-best in competitive situations?

If we want to develop a greater maturity in these areas, a good way to start is by listening patiently and considerately to the ideas of others. We can then begin to look more carefully at our interactions with others on a broader scale.

In any kind of relationship, two or more people are involved—not just ourselves. So we need to become willing to compromise when unanimity doesn't occur right away. This should be as true for simple day-to-day matters—choosing an evening's entertainment, for example—as for more serious issues.

We also should remind ourselves that we don't have to compete in *all* areas. And where competition is appropriate—sports, contests of skill, or career advancement—we should remember that it's better to compete with grace than with boorishness. After all, we can't always expect to be the best.

THOUGHT FOR TODAY: My way isn't always the right way.

April 24

Adversity introduces a man to himself.

—Anonymous

When I compare my life today with the way it used to be, it's hard to believe I'm describing the same person. In the past, I found it almost impossible to live life on life's terms. Most often, I dealt with adverse situations by sidestepping them or pretending they didn't exist. I was like a child who closes his eyes and imagines he is invisible.

But I wasn't playing a game. Because of my ongoing denial, unresolved and worsening problems erupted repeatedly. I despaired that things would never change.

Finally, somehow, one more time was one time too many. My defenses crumbled—pain and confusion forced me to ask for help. That's when my life began to change. Once I was able to seek and accept help, I found it in many places. I began to gradually reveal myself to others, benefiting greatly from their experiences. Most importantly, I began to include God in my life. And gradually, those once unresolvable problems became challenges offering growth-enhancing experience.

Looking back, I see that I have not only escaped from adversity, but have also been led into an entirely new dimension of living. I am the same person, to be sure, but I have gained new and life-fulfilling attitudes and perspectives.

THOUGHT FOR TODAY: Sometimes the "last straw" leads to the first taste.

A man may dwell so long upon a thought that it may take him prisoner.

—George Savile, Marquis of Halifax

What happens when we are obsessed? We become compulsively preoccupied with something, even to the point of insanity. An obsession, left unchecked, can affect us in ways ranging from emotional torment and physical illness to institutionalization and even death.

Just about anything can become an obsession—an unwanted thought, for example, or our reactions to people, places, or things. Although such matters vary from person to person, some obsessions—alcohol or other drugs, food, sex—are more serious than others and can, in fact, kill us.

But any obsession, no matter how seemingly harmless—cleanliness, exercise, compulsive punctuality—can cause great anguish. And because of the way they make us feel, these relatively innocuous obsessions can lead us back, as a means of escape, to more deadly ones.

How do we rid ourselves of obsessions? Long and painful experience at trying has taught us that we can't rid ourselves of them. We have found that God alone can remove obsessions, and that He will do so only when we have become entirely ready to have them removed.

THOUGHT FOR TODAY: God's power can relieve us of our obsessions—but only when we're ready.

April 26

When people are bored, it is primarily with their own selves that they are bored.

—Eric Hoffer

Along with its rewards, the recovery process entails many adjustments, especially at the beginning. When we are newly clean and sober, many of us have a problem with boredom, as one important example. This is hardly surprising, considering that our activities no longer revolve around our addictions. Besides that, we're in an entirely new state of consciousness; for the first time in years we have a true sense of time passing.

Reality is the same as it's always been—*we're* the ones who are changing. Therefore it doesn't take long to realize that overcoming boredom is our responsibility. It's up to us now to see what's out there—and to discover and develop our hidden talents, capabilities, and interests.

Those things we experienced under the influence of our addictions are so much more entertaining and exciting now that we're "there" to enjoy them. Some of us missed out on a decade or more of music, art, films, and books; in sobriety we're now able to renew our interest.

In a very short time, what at first seemed like a problem in our new life has turned into an unexpected bonanza. It's hard to believe that we were actually bored. Today, in fact, we sometimes wish we had more time to enjoy and appreciate our bountiful blessings.

THOUGHT FOR TODAY: Boredom is a state of mind that disappears when we take initiative.

To give up pretensions is as blessed a relief as to get them gratified.

—William James

If we are going to make real progress in seeking and doing God's will, we have to try to discard our pretensions along with our old ideas. First and foremost, we have to give up the pretense that self-sufficiency works. We should remember from our own hard lessons that we have little power insofar as most things are concerned, while God has all power.

We should strive also to be ourselves instead of masquerading as somebody we're not. We can do this by accepting our limitations, defining our capabilities, and going on from there—rather than continuing our pretense and getting nowhere.

If we find during these efforts that we have been spiritually pretentious, we should examine the motives behind our behavior. We might ask, for example, if we were trying to impress others by paying lip service to faith instead of living and practicing it. In this as well as all other areas of pretentiousness, we would do well to pray for the willingness to change and then humbly ask for God's help to become changed.

THOUGHT FOR TODAY: Spiritual pretentiousness fools no one and serves no one, least of all God.

April 28

We want facts to fit the preconceptions. When they don't it is easier to ignore the facts than to change the preconceptions.
—Jessamyn West

Of all my preconceptions, the one that was most damaging and limiting—the one that delayed my recovery from alcoholism more than any other—was my denial of God's existence. As a card-carrying atheist, I believed that people who put their faith in God had their heads in the clouds rather than in reality. I viewed them as fools and suckers, and that gave me a feeling of superiority. Besides, if there was a God, why was He ignoring *me*?

As I mumbled that it was a sign of weakness to depend on something so unscientific as a Higher Power, my health and sanity continued to deteriorate. Finally it was adamantly pointed out to me by a recovering alcoholic that since willpower had never worked, I could either face an alcoholic death or begin to live life on a spiritual basis—clearly not an easy choice for a lifelong atheist.

Needless to say I chose the latter course and was able to return to the world of the living. To my amazement and eventual great satisfaction, I gradually came to believe in a Power greater than myself. And I discovered through my own experience that, for me, dependence on God is the only true independence.

THOUGHT FOR TODAY: Discard your preconceptions, then face the facts.

The fountain of beauty is the heart, and every generous thought illustrates the walls of your chamber.

—Francis Quarles

Very few people are truly satisfied with their looks. We all gaze at our reflections from time to time and wish we were more attractive. By dwelling negatively on our appearances this way, we are being not only unfair but also unkind to ourselves.

When we pick apart the way we look, don't we usually judge ourselves unrealistically and exaggeratedly, as if we're standing before a fun house mirror? Aren't we comparing ourselves to media and cultural standards that concentrate on the exceptional outward beauty of a few?

We say that "beauty is only skin deep," yet many of us continue to place inordinate emphasis on our physical characteristics. If this is the case, perhaps it's time to focus seriously on the true beauty within, rather than paying mere lip service to the concept.

The most beautiful people are those whose spirit radiates outward. Their beauty is reflected in the way they think and act—in the way they treat others and view the world. Their inner beauty shines through not only in their faces, but in their entire philosophy of living.

THOUGHT FOR TODAY: True beauty resides in the heart and flows outward.

April 30

No man can tell another his faults so as to benefit him unless he loves him.

—Henry Ward Beecher

In our daily interactions we sometimes find it necessary to criticize other people for various reasons. Such confrontations are almost always difficult and unpleasant, and we tend to want to delay or avoid them. Yet they may be required.

The issue could be one of safety, where a person's actions are creating a dangerous situation. If someone's behavior has been affecting us adversely, it may be important that we state our case to achieve peace of mind. Or in the case of a close friendship, a confrontation may be required for the ongoing health and stability of the relationship.

When we feel it's necessary to take some action along these lines, it's best to think it through first. We should examine our motives to be sure we're not simply being mean-spirited and out to "get" someone, or that we're not "constructively criticizing" someone because of our own self-righteousness.

Finally, remembering that nobody likes to be criticized, we might put ourselves in the other person's shoes and try to make our points in a gentle and even loving way. If possible, we can offer helpful suggestions rather than simply describing what's "wrong." Later, when things get better, it can mean a lot to the other person if we mention the improvement.

THOUGHT FOR TODAY: If you must criticize, check the method as well as the motive.

Pride, like a magnet, constantly points to one object, self; unlike the magnet, it has no attractive pole, but at all points repels.

—Charles Caleb Colton

Many of us have to be reminded over and over that when we are filled with pride we are filled with self— and are therefore unable to rely on a Higher Power. One reason we have difficulty understanding the negative impact of pride is that for a long time we lived our lives believing that pride would pull us through.

Addicted people before recovery are often told, for example, by nonaddicted friends and family members that they have no willpower, that they're weak-willed, that they have no backbone. In our desperate state, anything makes sense, so we exert our wills even harder—in effect, battling self-centeredness with more "self"—which is not unlike trying to extinguish a fire by dousing it with gasoline.

The thing that finally brings us to our knees and into the gates of recovery is the realization that we have *no* power. In fact, lack of power was our dilemma. We have learned the hard way—which perhaps in these life and death matters is the best way—that God, who has all power, will exercise it on our behalf when He is sought.

THOUGHT FOR TODAY: God can and will if sought.

May 2

If God seems far away, who moved?

—Unknown

I once read a magazine article about a group of cloistered Benedictine nuns who devoted virtually every waking moment to prayer and meditation. They interrupted their practice of silence to be interviewed. The magazine reporter asked one of the nuns to describe, as specifically as she could, her relationship with God.

"It's like a relationship with anyone else," she replied with candor. "Sometimes it's pure bliss, and other times you wonder why you're in it at all."

Reading that article eased my mind and opened my eyes. Here was a person who had dedicated her entire life and very being to spiritual pursuits, yet even she found the path not always a smooth one.

In my own experience there have been times when I've felt remote from God. It's likely that there always will be such periods—when I feel that He's not there, that He's not listening, or even that He has abandoned me.

When I do feel like that, I can rest assured that it's only temporary, reminding myself that conscious contact will eventually be restored as long as I continue to seek Him.

THOUGHT FOR TODAY: We may not always feel God's presence, but He is always there.

They must often change who would be constant in happiness and wisdom.

—Confucius

We all tend to resist change, although few of us are willing to admit it. We find it easier to say that we're "set in our ways," or that "you can't teach an old dog new tricks." Even when the status quo in our jobs, relationships, or habits has become unsatisfactory or even painful, we may feel that the prospect of change is more frightening than what we're already enduring.

But feelings aren't facts. We need only look around us to see that change is usually beneficial, desirable, and necessary. If we take the time to think about nature, or the seasons—indeed, about life itself—we can become more comfortable with the idea of change and more able to accept it when it occurs.

Many of us have found that the most meaningful and rewarding changes are the ones that take place within ourselves. When we positively change our values and attitudes, for example, we are not only happier, but far less likely to be buffeted by outside forces. We discover, too, that while we can learn much from books and the experiences of others, true wisdom comes from our own experiences and our willingness to grow through change.

THOUGHT FOR TODAY: Seek change for the right reasons, rather than fear it for the wrong ones.

May 4

First say to yourself what you would be and then do what you have to do.

—Ralph Waldo Emerson

It's likely that our willful efforts to run the show resulted in damaged or destroyed relationships. Perhaps we're also carrying around guilt for things we've done in the past. When we try to clear away this damage by making amends, we embark on a sort of personal and spiritual housecleaning.

Even though we recognize the necessity of cleaning house, we may be reluctant to begin. Perhaps we don't want to remind people of our past behavior. We might be afraid they'll become angry or be unwilling to accept our amends.

When we express these concerns to our friends or spiritual advisers, they tell us that the reaction we get isn't important. Our goal is not to win the approval of others. We're reminded that we are really making amends for our own sake. We do so to rid ourselves of the guilt of past actions in order to live more comfortably today. Making amends to the people we have harmed can be one of the most difficult undertakings of our new life, but it can also provide us with some of the richest rewards.

THOUGHT FOR TODAY: Making amends helps *us* get on with the business of living.

The man is happiest who lives from day to day and asks no more, garnering the simple goodness of a life.

—Euripides

One of the easiest concepts to understand—yet one of the most difficult to apply—is living "a day at a time." It certainly isn't something we can accomplish immediately or ever practice with perfection.

When we first became aware of this age-old concept, we dismissed it as irrelevant to our lives. We grew up as goal setters who approached just about everything, from career objectives to relationships, in terms of forever. No other philosophy made sense to us.

What changed our minds? When we grew tired of constant frustration, of taking one step forward and two steps back, we finally became willing to try something new. We had seen that some of our friends achieved far more success in their endeavors, especially those requiring a lot of discipline, by undertaking them a day at a time instead of "for the rest of their lives." They were happy and comfortable; they were meeting challenges with grace rather than gritted teeth.

So we tried to live a day at a time in one small area—perhaps diet, or getting along with a difficult person. Because we found success, we became willing to apply the concept to other areas. And we learned to live a day at a time simply by trying each day to do so.

THOUGHT FOR TODAY: Enjoy your life a day at a time.

May 6

I care not so much what I am in the opinion of others as what I am in my own; I would be rich of myself, and not by borrowing.

—Michel Eyquem de Montaigne

Why do so many of us persist in judging ourselves harshly? Why don't we pay attention to the good things?

Part of it has to do with the familiarity of our distorted view of ourselves; we've grown accustomed to it. Some of us actually take comfort in the status quo because we're afraid to work on our poor self-image. Maybe we won't give ourselves a break because we're guilt-ridden—not only because of our own past actions, but also because of pressures created by the actions of family members.

What does it take to get out of this emotional rut? First, we have to be truly fed up with our self-inflicted suffering. We then need to make conscious and repeated efforts to reverse the self-image we've carried around for so long. One useful tool is periodically drawing up a list of character assets. In addition, when compliments come our way, we try to get into the habit of accepting them graciously rather than shrugging them off.

Some people find it most helpful, when they automatically attack themselves, to stop in mid-sentence or mid-thought and say aloud, "No, that's just not true."

THOUGHT FOR TODAY: A distorted self-image obscures the sunshine of life.

One's real life is often the life that one does not lead.
—Oscar Wilde

In a very real sense my negative attitudes and behavior kept me from living my own life. I spent so much time extricating myself from actual and imagined disasters that I relinquished the freedom to enjoy life as it unfolded.

I lived above my means both literally and figuratively, abusing expense accounts as well as the trust of my employers. The image I attempted to present to others differed greatly from the way I behaved and actually felt about myself. At least half of my time was spent trying to cover my tracks and alibi my way out of one or another misadventure.

Occasionally these days I tend to take my sobriety and serenity for granted. Gratitude comes in an overwhelming rush, however, when I think even momentarily of those hellish yesterdays.

I'm grateful that I'm no longer trapped in a web of deceit. I'm grateful that I can be honest and free in so many ways. I'm grateful that I don't have to pretend to be somebody else and can joyously lead my own real life.

THOUGHT FOR TODAY: True freedom is the freedom to be the real you.

May 8

Besides the noble art of getting things done, there is the noble art of leaving things undone. The wisdom of life consists in the elimination of non-essentials.

—Lin Yutang

Yesterday I had the best of intentions. I set out to get a lot done. I also intended to be kind and understanding, to take the time to pray and meditate, and to keep a firm grasp on my serenity no matter what.

The day turned out a lot differently than I expected. My attention was diverted and I put things off. I became upset and lashed out at a friend. I completely forgot about God. At the end I was not only disappointed and frustrated, but also annoyed at myself for falling short.

What can I do differently today to bridge the gap between my intentions and actions? First of all, I'll try to be certain that my intentions are not only well-defined, but also realistic. That way I won't set myself up to fail again. I'll also put first things first and organize my intentions by priority.

As the day unfolds, I'll try to be flexible and understanding when anything unexpected arises. And finally, I'll try to remember that I am but one person in a big world and can only do so much. I can't be all things to all people anymore than I can be all things to myself.

THOUGHT FOR TODAY: Your intentions for the day ahead can either be a solid foundation for accomplishment—or a ball and chain.

God is our refuge and strength, a very present help in trouble.
—Psalms 46:1

The most challenging circumstances of our lives often are those about which we can do absolutely nothing. We've already done everything that's possible; now all we can do is go about our business while we await an uncertain outcome.

This frequently happens during times of serious illness. Once we've gotten medical treatment and taken other necessary steps, we're utterly powerless. We have to step back and wait. Similarly, relationships sometimes require that one partner do his or her best to carry on while the other is incapable of doing so. Whether or not the marriage or partnership itself survives remains to be seen. The same is true during times of great financial stress, when we are challenged by the specter of possible bankruptcy or failure.

To relieve the burden during such periods, we can try to continue our normal routine. We can literally put one foot in front of the other, acting *as if* things will turn out as we hope. If the opposite occurs, at least we'll be in a better position to start again than if we had panicked or tried to escape in some way.

We can also use this time to strengthen our trust in God, remembering that He alone can provide us with endurance and calm strength for the long intervals of uncertainty that we cannot escape.

THOUGHT FOR TODAY: During periods of stressful uncertainty, act "as if" and try to carry on.

May 10

It is curious to note the old sea-margins of human thought.
Each subsiding century reveals some new mystery; we build
where monsters used to hide themselves.
—Henry Wadsworth Longfellow

Only after many years of confusion and resistance did spirituality become an integral part of my life. To this day I wouldn't presume to comprehend the dynamics of spiritual growth, but I do have a clearer picture of what seems to be taking place.

I gained knowledge of spiritual principles from books and by listening to others, and for quite some time that's as far as it went. Looking back, that knowledge remained useless until it penetrated to deeper levels— the levels of heart and soul.

It was only when knowledge gave way to understanding that my resistance diminished enough for me to start applying what I had learned. Admittedly, I did so at first with strong reservations. But results were quickly apparent, and that provided the impetus I needed to move on. When I tentatively tried to replace painful fear with reassuring faith, to recall one memorable turning point, I experienced relief that I had never imagined possible.

Beyond those first three phases of development— *knowledge, understanding,* and *application*—a fourth one is vital to my continued spiritual growth: to freely pass on to others what has been revealed and given to me.

THOUGHT FOR TODAY: First knowledge, then understanding, then application, then sharing.

If a man speaks or acts with pure thought, happiness follows him like a shadow that never leaves him.

—Buddha

As we become increasingly willing to live on a spiritual plane, our motives in many areas gradually change. In the past when we were charitable to others, for example, it was usually with the expectation of receiving something in return.

We frequently gave to others in order to look good and win their approval. We offered gifts as a way to gain control, or buy favors. We were generous out of a sense of obligation, or because we needed to get off the hook.

Now that we are progressing spiritually and taking actions to become free of self-centeredness and self-seeking, the path is growing narrower. We find that we want to—indeed, we must—be honest, aboveboard, and pure of motive in all our affairs. No longer can we get by with behavior disguised as one thing, yet calculated to achieve something else and benefit us in some way.

Today when we reach out to others, we do so unconditionally. Most often, we are motivated by a generosity of spirit. There are no strings attached to our actions. We are anxious to pass on those same gifts that God, through others, has so freely given to us—love, understanding, patience, and compassion.

THOUGHT FOR TODAY: Our motives speak more loudly than our words or actions.

May 12

Maturity: Among other things, not to hide one's strength out of fear and, consequently, live below one's best.
—Dag Hammarskjöld

A woman I know began to play tennis again after many years away from the sport. I asked her why she ever gave it up, considering how much she enjoys the game. She told me that she began to play in her teens.

"I was a natural," she recalled, "and when I played in a casual game I was fine. But I'd get totally psyched out in competition." Her self-consciousness in matches was so great that she choked her shots. At times her wrist wobbled uncontrollably.

"So I just quit," she said. "And then one day, maybe ten years later, I was watching these people playing tennis in a park. They were having a terrific time. I remembered how good I was, and I got really sad thinking about how my low self-esteem had caused me to quit."

The sadness was followed by a great awakening. It dawned on the woman that she had been sitting on the sidelines not only in tennis, but in virtually all areas of her life. "People around me were competing and winning. They were getting better jobs and having successful relationships, while I was still choking my shots and psyching myself out.

"I'm working on my serve and my backhand," she concluded. "But mostly I'm working on my insides. It's time for me to get back in the game, and I don't mean just tennis."

THOUGHT FOR TODAY: Don't let fear force you to the sidelines.

Few blame themselves until they have exhausted all other possibilities.

—Anonymous

What if we had the opportunity to somehow start all over again? What if we could actually erase everything in the past and present, and begin again with a clean slate? Things would be different this time around. We wouldn't make the same mistakes we made before. We'd have a chance to be really happy. Right?

It's always tempting to imagine that our problems will disappear if we run away from them. In fact, many of us have tried it on occasion. We've pulled up stakes and moved to different towns. We've abruptly ended relationships or begun new ones. We've changed careers. We've even tried altering our appearance in order to "solve" our problems.

The catch is, we can't run away from *ourselves*. No matter where we go or what we do, we take our perceptions, misconceptions, and old ideas with us.

What we learn over time, and through experience, is that most of our troubles come from our own attitudes and reactions—not from circumstances around us. We can transform our lives, but not by running away to new ones. We can do so only by changing from within.

THOUGHT FOR TODAY: The biggest problem is my reaction to the problem.

May 14

More dangers have deceived men than forced them.
—Francis Bacon

What's the most dangerous thing I could do today? Probably it would be to embrace again the old idea that I'm in charge—that I have power—that I can and should manage not only my own life, but the lives of everyone around me.

For years that idea totally deceived and almost destroyed me. Even though my addictions were fueled by self-will running riot, I believed that what I really needed was *more* willpower. I was able to begin my recovery only when I accepted a new idea: that I am in fact power*less*—that God alone has all power.

The dangerous and deceitful idea that I should be in charge is still rooted somewhere in my brain. Perhaps it always will be. But I've learned how to keep it from blooming, even though it remains powerful and patient.

If I continue to do the things that keep my faith strong—if I remember what I was, and remain grateful for what I've become, if I open my heart to others and listen when they open their hearts to me—then the old idea will remain just that.

THOUGHT FOR TODAY: Willpower has nothing to do with recovery.

Hating people is like burning down your house to get rid of a rat.

—Harry Emerson Fosdick

Hatred is an all-too-common human failing. Everyone knows what it's like to hate someone. Next time we feel hatred building up, let's try to remember what happens during an all-out explosion of this dangerous emotion.

When we hate someone, we are the ones who actually suffer. The person we hate is often totally unaware of our feelings, and in any case is unlikely to be affected at all, yet we experience real pain and unhappiness.

Our hatred can cause us to act irrationally; we may end up doing something we regret. Then the torment we already feel is compounded by feelings of guilt and remorse.

For a newly recovering person, an onslaught of this potent emotion can literally provide a push over the edge.

When we stop to think about the destructive potential of hatred, it quickly becomes obvious that we're dealing with a chain reaction emotion. Hatred not only consumes us, precluding rational thought or behavior, but it also interferes with our spirituality by blocking off our channel to God.

THOUGHT FOR TODAY: When we hate, we suffer.

May 16

Good actions are the invisible hinges on the doors of heaven.
—Victor Hugo

Today we want to remain self-aware and know we are right with the world. It's not enough anymore for us to just get by, allowing ourselves to be swept in and out of situations like a cork on the tide.

God has given us free will; He has blessed us with choices and capabilities. If we use our will rightly by aligning it with His will, our days will be more peaceful, productive, and satisfying. Each day it is possible to bring this intention into everything we do. The choice is ours.

In the morning we review our plans for the day. We ask God to show us the way, to guide our actions and thinking.

As our day progresses, we take the time to renew our conscious contact with God. We remind ourselves that we are not in charge.

At the day's end we look closely at our involvements and attitudes. We ask ourselves if we are carrying over anything that needs to be taken care of promptly. We express our gratitude to God for all His blessings.

THOUGHT FOR TODAY: God has blessed us with capabilities—and choices.

We don't get to know people when they come to us; we must go to them to find out what they are like.

—Goethe

As a teenager I once hitchhiked by myself across the United States. I remember being let off one night at a remote crossroads. Through the lighted windows of a farmhouse I could see a family seated around a dinner table. They were talking and laughing and seemed very happy.

I still recall my feelings at that moment. The house symbolized my life: I was on the outside looking in—I had no friends or even real acquaintances. Although I yearned for the warmth and camaraderie I saw through that window, I knew that I would never have it.

Looking back, I'm sure that even in those days people reached out to me in friendship. So low was my self-esteem, however, that I shut them out in fear of what they might find.

Had anyone suggested even jokingly during those painful years that someday I would not only fit in, but be literally surrounded by true friends, I would have felt they were mocking me. But thanks to God, that is today's miraculous reality. I freely allow people to come to me, and frequently I reach out to discover what they are like. Instead of the ache of alienation, I am now filled with a deep sense of belonging.

THOUGHT FOR TODAY: You can reach out beyond your *self* by reaching out to another.

May 18

Happiness does not lie in happiness, but in the achievement of it.

—Fëdor Mikhailovitch Dostoevski

One of our most common misconceptions is the belief that happiness depends on luck—some people have it, but most people don't. Carrying the idea further, many people believe they'll be happy if they meet Mr. or Miss Perfect, if they win the lottery, if they're in the right place at the right time and get the right job, and so on.

As we go through life we learn that nothing could be further from the truth. Although luck may play some part in meeting a person you like, finding a special job, or even achieving financial success—none of these things guarantees happiness. Mr. or Miss Perfect can easily become Mr. or Miss Bad News. If it turns out we're not suited for that special job, we can quickly become miserable. And financial good fortune can just as often cause problems as pleasure.

True happiness, we find, comes in large measure from our willingness to work for it. It comes from a job well done, from helping others, and from doing the things that make us feel good about ourselves. The reality is that each of us is responsible for his or her own happiness.

THOUGHT FOR TODAY: Happiness is an inside job.

We never know how high we are—till we are called to rise.
—Emily Dickinson

We're often told that "the road gets narrower" as we continue our spiritual journey. This describes our efforts to understand and apply the concepts we have learned at ever-deeper levels. Especially challenging in this regard is the goal of becoming less selfish and self-seeking.

Sometimes we may feel that we're making unsatisfactory progress in this area. That's understandable, for it is all but impossible to mentally measure one's progress as it relates to matters of "self." From time to time, however, God places us in situations that allow us to clearly see how far we've actually come. Following such experiences, we realize we've made more progress than we think we have.

Typically, for example, we find ourselves in the midst of a family crisis. Everyone is distraught and exhausted; no one has any idea what to do. To our surprise, we realize that we no longer have a need to self-seekingly "take" from the situation as we so often did in the past. Instead we're anxious to provide support, solace, and solutions. We're able to be caring and useful because our personal needs are being met elsewhere, in more positive and constructive ways.

THOUGHT FOR TODAY: Our spiritual progress is better measured by our actions than our thoughts.

Look well into thyself; there is a source of strength which will always spring up if thou wilt always look there.
—Marcus Aurelius

It was only after I had gained some degree of spiritual enlightenment that I realized the extent to which dependency ruled my life. I depended on others for security, approval, and prestige. These were not simply emotional requirements on my part; they were out-and-out demands.

Moreover, I wasn't satisfied unless these demands were fulfilled according to my exact specifications. Not surprisingly, I was constantly disappointed. Some people in this situation become frustrated, angry, and rebellious; others become depressed and withdrawn.

I wasn't aware of it at the time, but by demanding that my inner needs be fulfilled by other people, I put myself on the emotional chopping block time and time again.

For most of our lives we have thought the problem was our anger, rebelliousness, or depression. But we've since discovered that these reactions were but symptoms that masked the *real* problem—our inappropriate emotional dependencies.

Today we are convinced that our need for security and emotional well-being cannot be provided by people, places, or things. It can only come from within ourselves and from God.

THOUGHT FOR TODAY: I gain emotional security by decreasing my dependence on others and increasing my dependence on God.

To be alive, to be able to see, to walk, to have houses, music, paintings—it's all a miracle. I have adopted the technique of living life from miracle to miracle.

—Artur Rubinstein

There was a time in my life when I would scoff at the very idea of miracles. Which is not to say that on certain occasions I didn't hope desperately that something miraculous would come to pass. If I could get rid of my hangover by taking a few drinks—without getting drunk all over again—that would have been a miracle. If I could only get bailed out, get to the airport on time, and make my deadline—that would be a miracle.

Out of the true miracle of my sobriety today flows a host of other miracles. I am the same person I was back then, to be sure, but I feel far differently about myself. My self-loathing has been replaced with a sense of self-respect and usefulness.

There are days when I am literally astonished to be alive. When I think back to the constantly perilous existence I led—and to the times I was close to death—I am filled with gratitude just to be breathing, let alone to have physical and mental capabilities.

Today I am aware that all of this has come to pass only because of the power and grace of God. That awareness, for me, is perhaps the greatest miracle of all.

THOUGHT FOR TODAY: Expect a miracle, accept a miracle.

A good action is never lost; it is a treasure laid up and guarded for the doer's need.

—Pedro de la Barca Calderon

We're comfortable because everything is going smoothly; we've truly never had it so good. Moreover, we're convinced that our success is a direct result of God's presence in our lives, for we surely couldn't have done it on our own.

Yet ironically, this is the time when some of us slack off on our spiritual activities and interactions with others. We cut down and stop doing the things that got us where we are today.

Perhaps we don't pray, meditate, or express our gratitude to God as often as we used to. We may begin to lose touch with those who have been so helpful to us from the beginning. We may feel we "don't have enough time" to reach out to others.

Of course, it's easier to be willing to do these things when we're struggling and having difficulty. We've found, however, that nothing pays off like *consistency* in spiritual activity; we can continue to grow spiritually no matter what our circumstances.

Besides that, why should we shortchange ourselves when times are good? This is when we have the opportunity to make large deposits in our "spiritual bank." We can build up an account of strength and God-consciousness that will be available when we need to draw on it.

THOUGHT FOR TODAY: Spiritual activity is just as necessary and rewarding during good times as it is during difficult times.

Fanaticism consists of redoubling your effort when you have forgotten your aim.

—George Santayana

We all know how tormenting obsessions can be. They cause mental anguish and can completely disrupt our lives. We can become so obsessed with an expected phone call, for example, that we imprison ourselves in our homes. We can become so obsessed with the new computer at work that we end up putting in eighteen-hour days.

Obsessions also can lead to fanatical behavior. We may find ourselves "playing spy" because of our obsessive relationship with another person. We may even be tempted to take an ax to that new computer.

From experience we've learned that the only way to become free of an obsession is to ask God to remove it. This is the one thing that works—we know that. But we also know that it sometimes takes time before God relieves our obsessions.

Waiting can be very painful, but there are things we can do to help ourselves. Each time the obsession surfaces, we can make a conscious and disciplined effort to center our thoughts on God. We can also talk with another person about our obsessions, and we can write about them. We can try to stay busy.

Most important, when we pray for the obsession to be removed, we can also pray for patience and faith that it will be removed.

THOUGHT FOR TODAY: Take the power away from your obsession by centering your thoughts on God.

May 24

Our grand business in life is not to see what lies dimly at a distance, but to do what lies clearly at hand.

—Thomas Carlyle

One of the hardest things for any of us to do is to end a relationship. This can be true whether the tie is romantic or with an employer, friend, or family member. For various reasons, we often remain in damaging relationships long after we realize it's time to move on.

We may fear being alone. We may be unable or reluctant to face changes and the pain of letting go. Perhaps our sense of obligation to a person is based on guilt; for one reason or another, we feel we "owe" them.

Because of our improving self-worth, we're less willing to stay in unhealthy and damaging relationships these days. We believe that we deserve better. We're learning to honestly evaluate our ties with others, putting aside rationalizations and looking at the reality. We try to focus on the way things are right now, rather than how they used to be or could be in the future.

We ask ourselves if the benefits of staying in the relationship outweigh the consequences of doing so. Although we may feel hooked into a situation because someone "needs" us, we also have to consider our own needs, by asking, "What's best for my well-being?"

THOUGHT FOR TODAY: I'm unwilling to put up with damaging relationships; I deserve better.

The wind in a man's face makes him wise.

—John Ray

The way we react to disappointments can often be more painful and debilitating than the actual events. Some people, for example, miss out on the joys of life because they never get over disappointments. They actually become immobilized by their bitterness and cynicism. Others burden themselves with long-lasting resentment against those who supposedly let them down or spurned them. Still other people withdraw to lick their wounds, refusing to trust anyone ever again.

Major disappointments can be personally tragic, there's no question about that. However, we *don't* have to go to the aforementioned extremes. In most instances we have choices.

Let's remind ourselves first that life has to go on—and *will* go on—in spite of adversity and our subsequent disappointment. Let's make every effort to learn from the event and to accept things the way they are right now. If we can do that, it will be much easier to make new plans and develop new strategies in line with our changed situations. Most important, we can seek comfort in our faith, trusting in God's wisdom and the rightness of His plan for us.

THOUGHT FOR TODAY: Everything happens for a reason, in accordance with the plan of a loving God.

May 26

To stand on one leg and prove God's existence is a very different thing from going down on one's knees and thanking Him.
—Sören Kierkegaard

I once heard a man say that his consciousness of the presence of God had become the most important fact in his life. The statement made a strong impression on me. It seemed at the time that the man was "saintly" in some way; certainly it would be impossible for me ever to feel as he did.

I had "believed" in God for a relatively short time, evolving from hostile atheism to holier-than-thou agnosticism. That is, I accepted the idea of God but denied the possibility of knowing Him or of being known by Him. In any event my beliefs were inconsequential, since I made no effort to actually include God in my life. Rather, I prided myself on being self-sufficient.

I looked good on the outside, as they say, but had begun to feel an emptiness within. Life seemed meaningless, lacking direction or a sense of real joy.

It's difficult to describe what happened soon afterward. Suffice it to say that I underwent a profound spiritual experience. In spite of my vaunted self-sufficiency, I humbly asked for God's help.

Now I too have come to believe that the consciousness of God's presence is the most important fact in my life. Today, in prayer and through service to others, I thank Him for my life, for my sanity, and for showing me the way.

THOUGHT FOR TODAY: You can best thank God through service to others.

A great part of courage is the courage of having done the thing before.

—Ralph Waldo Emerson

One of the realities many of us must deal with in early recovery is our immaturity. Our social, emotional, and even intellectual development often slowed considerably or stopped when we began drinking or using drugs addictively. Some of us missed out on learning the skills that could later enable us to be comfortable and confident in demanding situations—such as job interviews. Others never had the opportunity to learn such basics as dating, making friends, or simply carrying on a conversation with another person.

When we begin to recover and face the real world without our "medicine," we are confronted with a variety of unfamiliar and often painful emotions and challenges. Even simple tasks are often difficult: shopping for clothes, ordering food in restaurants, even going through supermarket check-out lines.

Just because we temporarily lack certain skills or the experience necessary to develop them, that's no reason to feel ashamed, foolish, or "less than." Invariably we find that we can quickly acquire both the skills and the experience—and can soon function in the world without limitation. What is more, as we become comfortable with ourselves and the world around us, we realize that we are not unique and need not face these challenges alone.

THOUGHT FOR TODAY: Addiction is progressive, but so is recovery.

May 28

The iron chain and silken cord are both equally bonds.
   —Johann Cristoph Friedrich von Schiller

A friend of mine tells a story about baby elephants. In countries where elephants are used as working animals, they must be trained when they are very young and not yet too powerful. The first thing a trainer does is fasten a heavy manacle and chain to the baby elephant's leg, securing the other end of the chain to a metal stake driven deep into the ground. When the elephant tries to walk freely about, it cannot move any farther than the end of the chain. Although the animal may try repeatedly to escape, it is held in check by its unyielding restraint.

After a period of time, the baby elephant stops testing the strength of the chain. It remains within the circle's limited circumference, completely passive. It has become thoroughly convinced that it cannot escape.

At that point the elephant can be used in the field and easily transferred from one location to another without concern. All it takes to hold the animal, despite its enormous strength, is a light rope and thin wooden stake. Because once the baby elephant has been conditioned in this manner, he remains convinced for the rest of his life that what was once true will always be true.

Have I begun to get rid of my baby elephant ideas?

THOUGHT FOR TODAY: It's never too soon or too late to change our convictions.

We are more often frightened than hurt; and we suffer more from imagination than from reality.

—Seneca

For many years I assumed that almost everything occurring in my self-centered little universe—from one person's whispered remark to another's sidelong glance—had to do with me personally. Considering the fact that I had zero self-esteem, it was ironic that I imagined the world revolving around me.

Yet my hypersensitivity to the actions of others caused me extreme pain. It was as if my emotional antennae picked up signals on some special frequency—one that most people didn't even know existed. My problem was compounded because I also reacted intensely to the pain of others, often absorbing it as if it were my own.

When I began my new life, a friend suggested that I put on an "invisible raincoat." This, she said, would temporarily shield me from unwelcome "vibes" while I learned more realistic and long-term solutions to my hypersensitivity. By taking actions that at first seemed unrelated to my problem, I gradually was able to counteract my self-centeredness while becoming more secure and self-assured.

While I'm still fine-tuned to the world around me, my reactions these days are far different. My sensitivity has been transformed from a painful liability into a positive force in my life.

THOUGHT FOR TODAY: Your emotional antennae can be redirected for positive reception.

May 30

Live each day as if your life had just begun.

—Goethe

Is this all there is? Is this it? Every one of us asks this question from time to time. We look at our lives and what's around us with the sense that there's nothing new and never will be. And because of this mood we probably feel disillusioned or even depressed. We experience the "same old things" in the "same old way."

Needless to say, this state of mind has nothing to do with what life actually has to offer. It has everything to do with our attitude—with the way we view the world and react to it. If we choose to see things only in shades of gray, that's what we're sure to experience. It's as simple as that.

If on the other hand we approach the day with a sense of wonder and interest, it's likely that we'll experience things far differently. If we have a receptive attitude rather than fixed and cynical expectations, we greatly increase our potential to be enthusiastic, inspired, and fulfilled.

In its own special way, each day offers an endless variety of experience, excitement, and opportunity. On every level the world is filled with wonders—it's all there. In the end, however, it's up to us. Our attitudes determine what we get out of life.

THOUGHT FOR TODAY: Today may seem to be the same as yesterday, but you have the opportunity to experience it in an entirely different way.

Be great in act, as you have been in thought. Suit the action to the word, and the word to the action.

—William Shakespeare

In order to further our progress, we try to apply spiritual principles in all our endeavors and relationships. Sometimes, though, we unwittingly practice these principles selectively. We act one way in the outside world, and another way when we are with those we love the most. Why do we do this? Why would we want to?

If we carefully and honestly examine our behavior, we may find that at times we have self-seeking motives. Perhaps we're kind, patient, and understanding in the outside world in order to get approval, to win favors, or simply to be accepted.

We may not do this to the same extent at home because we don't need to—that is, we already have the love and acceptance of our family, and frequently take them for granted. Besides, isn't it easier to practice principles such as self-restraint with outsiders than with those we know intimately?

If we sense that we have a double standard following a review of our behavior, it's probably time to get our motives and priorities back in order. For if we truly want to progress spiritually, we can't allow ourselves to be selective in *when*, *where*, or *why* we practice spiritual principles.

THOUGHT FOR TODAY: God has no double standard in offering His love.

June 1

Time cools, time clarifies; no mood can be maintained quite unaltered through the course of hours.

—Thomas Mann

We don't often think of time as being an active and essential part of the solutions to our problems. If we do think about time at all, we notice that "it flies," "it drags," or that we've wasted it. Summer approaches before we've realized that winter has ended. There's much more to time, however, than minutes, days, and weeks ticking away.

Time allows us to eventually accept conditions that, at the time of their original development, were wholly unacceptable.

Time also enables us to see things more clearly and put them into perspective. How often have we looked back at a once-bewildering situation and, from the vantage point of time and distance, been able to finally understand it?

Certainly time cools anger and tempers resentment. Even if we stubbornly refuse to seek and apply other solutions, time by itself can defuse explosive emotions. During periods of pain, moreover, time combined with previous experience assures us that "this too shall pass."

Although profound positive changes in attitudes and behavior can sometimes occur "overnight," such miraculous happenings are the exceptions. Most such changes take place gradually, and again time is a vital ingredient.

THOUGHT FOR TODAY: Time is on your side.

Let every soul be subject unto the higher powers, for there is no power but of God.

—Romans 13:1

When we finally concede to our innermost selves that we are powerless over other people, we begin to experience a new dimension of personal freedom. We become free of the emotional shackles that have destructively bound us to our addicted spouses, children, or dear friends. Where before we had been obsessed with trying to "fix" those we loved, we now are free to step aside—to lovingly release them into God's hands.

Unfortunately, others close to us—who have been similarly affected by addicted loved ones—aren't always able to find solutions. Typically, for example, one parent becomes willing to understand, accept, and apply spiritual solutions to her relationship with an addicted child. The other parent continues to react with frustration and impotent rage, even to the point of turning against his spouse and demanding, "How can you let our child destroy her life?"

As the spiritually enlightened parent in this example, we have to remember that we are as powerless over our tormented spouse as we are over our addicted child. All we can do is offer the same solutions that have brought freedom to us, realizing of course that we can't force acceptance or even understanding of those solutions.

THOUGHT FOR TODAY: Spiritual enlightenment may come to each of us at different times, but never too early or too late.

June 3

The actions of men are like the index of a book; they point out what is most remarkable in them.

—Heinrich Heine

I used to think that if only I could be smarter, more successful, or richer, I would most certainly be happier. Because of those misguided aspirations, the people I looked up to were the ones with money, property, and prestige.

Now that my values and attitudes have changed, the people I admire most include those who unobtrusively go about helping others. By watching the ways in which they reach out—the manner in which they share their experience, strength, and hope—I now understand what is meant by the expression, "God works through people."

That understanding has come to mean a great deal, for it is often difficult for me to know God's will. I've learned that I really can't go wrong, however, if I think of myself as a channel for His work, taking action to help others as I have been helped.

When I humbly reach out to another person with an offer of assistance, a word of encouragement, a compliment—or simply a warm smile—I find I'm the one who benefits most.

THOUGHT FOR TODAY: God works through people.

The worst sorrows in life are not its losses and misfortunes, but its fears.

—A. C. Benson

Only by carefully examining our fears can we realize how extensively they affect our lives. By holding us back from pursuing important goals—from doing what we otherwise might—fear often causes sorrows and regrets.

For example, if we're afraid of people, we tend to exclude them from our lives in various ways. We then miss out on their friendship and the special opportunity to learn new things from others.

Fear holds many of us back from advancement in the job arena. We may know with certainty that we deserve a raise or promotion, but fear of confrontation prevents us from stating our case. Instead, we accept what is actually unacceptable and wait with frustration until we are "noticed."

Or perhaps it's time to make a career change. Here again, we're immobilized by fear of failure. Consequently, we don't take the first step, and as a result resentfully continue to perform tasks that we've long since outgrown.

Am I still being held back from life's joyful experiences by fear? Or have I become willing to begin again by replacing fear with faith and taking small risks?

THOUGHT FOR TODAY: Reasoned risks are not to be feared.

June 5

In quietness and in confidence shall be your strength.
—Isaiah 30:15

Why do we meditate? It's a way to communicate with God—to establish and strengthen conscious contact with Him. Looking at it another way, meditation allows us to understand and map out our spiritual objectives before we try to move toward them.

Some people think that special skills are required before one can meditate, but that isn't the case at all. When we remember the purpose of meditation, it becomes clear how simple it can be. We meditate to open ourselves and receive guidance from God—and receiving is one of the functions our minds perform best. So we don't need to be at any particular spiritual level before we can meditate, nor do we need special knowledge or training.

The point is, anyone can meditate. It's a personal adventure, something each of us approaches in his or her own way. Meditation certainly shouldn't be viewed as a chore—it should be approached instead with enthusiasm and an openness to being inspired.

Soon after we begin to practice meditation regularly, we find that it is not at all "abstract," but, to the contrary, immensely practical. For it is from meditation that we gain knowledge of God's will for us. When we convert that knowledge into action, the rewards of meditation become abundantly evident and concrete.

THOUGHT FOR TODAY: Through meditation, we open ourselves to God's inspiration and guidance.

Whenever you have seen God pass, mark it, and go and sit in that window again.

—Henry Ward Beecher

Meditation is a spiritual practice that has enriched the lives of countless people throughout the centuries. It is neither mysterious, difficult, nor circumscribed by rules. In fact, no two individuals meditate in exactly the same manner; there are as many ways to meditate as there are people seeking God's guidance.

It is often said that we get out of meditation what we put into it. In other words, the spirit with which we try to improve our conscious contact with God is far more important than the form that we use. It's not that we ignore form, or method, but simply that we do what brings us the most desirable experience. Once a particular approach has been successful, we "sit in that window again."

When you begin to practice meditation, here are some ideas worth considering. In a place free of disturbing influences, try to be as relaxed and free of strain as possible. Let your mind rest. Strive to be less conscious of your body, thoughts, and surroundings—of everything but God.

Concentrate your attention on God rather than "nothing." Try to reflect on the nature of His love, wisdom, and power. Imagine His presence. Most important, approach your meditation with an expectant attitude, anticipating that you will receive inspiration and guidance from God.

THOUGHT FOR TODAY: Meditation has no limitations—neither of form nor of results.

June 7

Some people are always grumbling that roses have thorns; I am thankful that thorns have roses.

—Alphonse Karr

When people told me to "have a nice day" or "put on a happy face," I used to get really annoyed. I hated those meaningless clichés, whether they were in advice from other people, in songs, or on cocktail napkins.

I reacted as I did because of the way I had become accustomed to living. If someone had said to me, "Take time to smell the roses," chances are I wouldn't have understood what he or she meant. In fact, if I had stopped frowning down at the ground long enough to see the roses, it's likely I would have complained that they "attract insects."

Needless to say, I was damaged by such attitudes, and not always in obvious ways. Because I saw everything negatively, I was constantly angry. By the expression on my face, my comments, and my body language, I gave off negative energy that kept people away from me. I had no friends.

Now that my way of thinking has changed, those expressions that used to seem so trite have taken on real meaning in my life. I've learned that when I "accentuate the positive," I truly can "have a nice day."

THOUGHT FOR TODAY: Your attitude can turn today around—for better or for worse.

It is of immense importance to learn to laugh at ourselves.
—Katherine Mansfield

We have learned that pride is the essence of self-importance, and we have gradually become aware of the many ways in which this character defect has injured us. One of the main thrusts of our new life is to become free of self and thus gain greater humility.

We're making steady progress. Our growing humility is allowing us to rely more on God. Because our pride has diminished and we're less filled with self, we don't need to take ourselves as seriously as we used to.

In the past our slightest mistakes could cause us to become furious at ourselves. If someone teased us even mildly, we couldn't handle it. Nothing was minor; everything was major. Because we were so prideful, we were constantly on the defensive.

These days, in contrast, we have a far more accurate perspective of the way we fit into the world. We no longer feel compelled to blow ourselves out of proportion. It's so much easier to get along with others. Today we can laugh at ourselves, and what a relief that is!

THOUGHT FOR TODAY: When you take yourself too seriously, you put on an emotional straitjacket.

June 9

The good displeases us when we have not yet grown up to it.
—Nietzsche

As suffering addicts our lives were in perpetual crisis. Some of us were in and out of jails and hospitals. If we weren't being admitted to an institution, we were being discharged or bailed out. At home and at work our relationships were in constant turmoil. We were forever getting in trouble or trying to get out of it.

When we finally threw in the towel and began our recovery, our lives changed dramatically. But although we were out of immediate danger, we still found ourselves living from crisis to crisis. We were constantly stirred up.

We saw that other recovering addicts were living relatively trouble-free lives, and wondered what we were doing wrong. When we asked for help, the answer came quickly: Even though we had given up our life-threatening addictions, we were still hooked on "adrenaline." We had grown so used to living in crisis that we were unwittingly creating it for ourselves, making mountains out of molehills on a daily basis.

At first it was hard to see that we were responsible for causing our own turmoil. But soon we were able to acknowledge what we were doing. From then on we were usually able to rein ourselves in, instead of galloping headlong toward a new adrenaline "rush" of our own making.

THOUGHT FOR TODAY: If my life is in constant crisis, it may be because I'm hooked on adrenaline.

Love is an act of faith, and whoever is of little faith is also of little love.

—Erich Fromm

We thought we knew all about love, but actually we knew and understood very little. Over the years we developed many misconceptions about love, patterning our ideas and actions more on outside influences than on inner knowledge.

We looked forward to "falling" in love. When we met the right person, we expected love to bloom and endure automatically, without any effort on our part. All too often we confused love with infatuation or lust.

It was not until we began to build a relationship with God that we were able to understand and experience real love. Through our growing faith we learned about trust, acceptance, self-honesty, and generosity. We came to realize that God's love for us is unconditional, and that He will continue to care for us no matter what.

As we strengthened our relationship with God, success grew in other relationships. We had been learning about love without even realizing it. The trust, acceptance, honesty, and generosity we have acquired during our spiritual quest now benefits us in all areas of our lives. Today we realize that in order to have successful, loving relationships we must continue to employ these qualities at ever deeper levels.

THOUGHT FOR TODAY: As our faith deepens, so does our capacity to understand and experience real love.

June 11

Mere survival is an affliction. What is of interest is life, and the direction of that life.

—Guy Frégault

A familiar wall poster shows a kitten dangling by its front paws from an exercise bar. The kitten's fur is standing straight out and its eyes are filled with terror. The headline reads, "Hang in there, baby!"

Although the poster remains popular, I can't relate at all anymore to the philosophy it expresses. Yet in the past, I identified completely with that terror-stricken animal—because that's the way I used to live. Day after day I hung on by my fingernails. I fully expected that I would have to white-knuckle my way through life.

Today I know with certainty that I don't have to live that way anymore. I no longer believe that it's my destiny to "just get by," or that "life is hard and then you die."

I've learned from my own experience that just the opposite can be true—if I remain honest and open-minded, and if I'm willing to use the unfailingly effective spiritual tools that are always within reach. One of my deepest beliefs these days is that God truly wants me to enjoy my life—to be happy, free, and fulfilled.

THOUGHT FOR TODAY: You don't have to white-knuckle your way through life.

Fire that is closest kept burns most of all.
—William Shakespeare

All of us have done things and felt things that caused us embarrassment and guilt—even as memories. They became deep and painful secrets. But we resolved to live with them, despite the fact that they continued to eat away at us.

We realize now that by drawing a veil over our previous actions and feelings we were doing ourselves a serious disservice. Our secrets remained closed up within us, to the extent that we couldn't leave the past behind and get on with our lives. We stopped growing and, for a long time, suffered with an out-of-date self-image.

Eventually we learned that the best way to remove the power from our secrets was to divulge them completely to another person. We chose someone we trusted—a spiritual adviser, family member, or professional who would be understanding as well as discreet.

When we found the courage to take this liberating step, we experienced a tremendous sense of relief. Many of us finally were able to forgive ourselves and this, in turn, opened the door to still greater freedom. Soon our self-image caught up with the reality of our lives today; for the first time in years, we could respect ourselves.

THOUGHT FOR TODAY: By unburdening ourselves of our secrets, we can bring our self-image up to date.

June 13

We must always change, renew, rejuvenate ourselves; otherwise we harden.

—Goethe

From time to time we hear about people making sudden and drastic changes in their lives in response to major trauma. A heart attack, for example, precipitates long-delayed soul-searching, which leads to a career change or new life-style. Similarly, an unexpected divorce or the loss of a loved one leads to a complete reordering of priorities.

When such crisis-triggered metamorphoses work out for our friends or relatives, we're happy for them. But what about ourselves? Must we also be hit over the head with a sledgehammer before we're able to break out of rigid molds or stultifying patterns? Why does it have to take a catastrophe to spur us to action?

The point is that we can make these decisions anytime. God expects us to change. That's why we seek His guidance; that's why He has given us the power of choice and free will.

Once we become willing to make major changes, it can be frightening to take those first steps. But that's where our partnership with God comes into play again. He will always be there to guide and protect us. He will always provide us with the courage and strength we need to carry out His will in our own best interest.

THOUGHT FOR TODAY: We don't have to experience blindness to become willing to see the light.

The end of doubt is the beginning of repose.

—Petrarch

As a sort of last-gasp form of denial, some alcoholics in early recovery very carefully compare their drinking patterns with those of other alcoholics. Because they're still having trouble admitting that they are alcoholics, they come up with all sorts of rationalizations to "prove" that they are not: "I didn't drink hardly anything compared to those people." "I never drank before five o'clock." "I drank only good stuff."

The fallacy in all of this, of course, is that the common denominator among alcoholics is not how much you drink or what you drink, but what it does to you. Alcoholism is not only a physical addiction, but a mental obsession. Even if an alcoholic is not actively drinking, he or she can be so preoccupied with the idea of it that life becomes a nightmare. In fact, drinking itself is but a symptom of the underlying causes of this progressive, incurable, and often fatal disease.

But unlike other incurable diseases, alcoholism can be arrested. The first step in recovery is overcoming denial, conceding without reservation that one is indeed an alcoholic. Once this happens, an alcoholic can become willing to listen for similarities in feelings, rather than differences in drinking patterns.

THOUGHT FOR TODAY: It's not how much you drink or use, but how it affects you and your life.

June 15

It is impossible for a man to despair who remembers that his Helper is omnipotent.

—Jeremy Taylor

If at any time today I feel anxious, confused, or alone, I will remind myself that wherever I am, God is. Whether I am at work, at home, or traveling, God will protect and care for me. It doesn't matter whether I am intensely busy or simply relaxing; since His loving presence surrounds me, I am safe at all times.

Prayer is my access to God's strength and guidance. As I establish conscious contact with Him during the day, I will receive reassurance and peace. He will keep me from harm and also protect me from my own self-destructive tendencies. So long as I turn to God, I will be free from fear, anxiety, and the torment of indecision.

Am I unduly concerned about the behavior or well-being of a loved one? Do I fear that a certain situation, place, or person is somehow beyond the realm of God's protection? If such apprehensions begin to gnaw at me, I will decrease their power by focusing intently on the limitless scope of His power. I will again become reassured that this is God's world, and that His mantle of protection is all-encompassing.

THOUGHT FOR TODAY: God is present everywhere, so we can feel protected and secure all the time, in all places.

Search thy own heart; what paineth thee in others in thyself may be.

—John Greenleaf Whittier

When we are judgmental of others, we often focus on the very qualities we dislike in ourselves. It isn't easy to recognize and acknowledge this truth. And that's probably a primary reason why we're judgmental in the first place: When our eyes are turned outward, we're able to avoid looking at ourselves.

Yet if we honestly examine our judgments—if we take the time to think carefully about the things we find offensive in others—it's possible to learn much about our own faults.

When we see someone as pompous and a "blow-hard," aren't we able to quickly identify those characteristics because we've been that way ourselves? If we become annoyed at a friend's constant complaining, isn't it probably because we too often have had our own private "pity party"?

Unfortunately, we can continue to be judgmental of others for a relatively long time, because such behavior harms us only gradually and not very obviously. Slowly but surely, however, an erosion occurs; we become less understanding, tolerant, compassionate, and helpful.

In order to avoid harming others and myself, will I try to notice qualities I admire—instead of searching for ones I can dislike?

THOUGHT FOR TODAY: When we focus on the faults of others, we're able to avoid looking at our own.

167

June 17

The greatest mistake you can make in life is to be continually fearing you will make one.

—Elbert G. Hubbard

For years we insisted that our way was the right way—the only way. When things didn't work out, we rarely acknowledged our mistakes. For some of us, making a mistake meant "getting caught," and we went to great lengths to cover our mistakes with alibis, denial, and outright lies. Needless to say, even slight errors usually turned into big deals.

Thankfully, we don't have to live like that anymore. For our own sakes, we try to be honest and aboveboard in everything we do. As a result, we have nothing to hide or alibi. When we make a mistake these days, it's just that—a mistake. And since we no longer have to make such big deals of our mistakes, we're no longer afraid of making them.

More and more we're able to accept ourselves—our fallibility and limitations as well as our capabilities and potential for continued growth. We no longer feel compelled to punish ourselves for trivial errors, missteps, or misjudgments. We're learning to be more patient and gentle with ourselves.

THOUGHT FOR TODAY: Be human; give up the need to be perfect.

Everybody needs his memories. They keep the wolf of insignificance from the door.

—Saul Bellow

I awakened one morning filled with a profound sense of gratitude. During the night I had dreamed vividly about my life as it used to be. I had been returned to a particular July day when my despair and suicidal actions brought me to the brink of death.

Reflecting upon my life as it is today, I sat up in bed and thought, "I almost missed all of this."

Had I continued my descent into hell, I would have missed the sights, the sounds, and fragrances of the world as it finally became unveiled for me. I would have missed the opportunities of travel, books, films, music, and new experiences of infinite variety.

Had I not surrendered, I would have missed the warmth and reassurance of unconditional love and true friendship—the countless occasions to freely give and receive.

I would have missed the chance to know my true self, to discover my capabilities and limitations, to replace self-hatred with self-love.

Above all, I would have missed the joyous awareness of God's presence in my life, and the comfort and security of His love. Without His grace I assuredly would have missed it all.

THOUGHT FOR TODAY: Fear can be replaced with faith, hopelessness with wholeness, despair with joy.

June 19

I was shipwrecked before I got aboard.

—Seneca

The way we look at things and react to them—in short, our attitudes—can greatly influence our experiences. Everybody knows that. We sometimes forget, though, that our attitudes tend to spill over into other parts of our lives and the lives of others.

Let's say your cousin is getting married and you've been invited to the wedding. You don't want to go, mostly because you resent someone in the wedding party. Because of your attitude, everything becomes a chore, from choosing a gift to deciding what to wear. Prior to the event, your negativity taints everything you do. At the wedding you have an awful time. Your sulking is obvious to your cousin, who takes it personally. For a long time afterward you regret your behavior.

Of course, it doesn't have to be that way. You can make a sincere effort to change your attitude and "rewrite" the entire scenario.

You're happy for your cousin and her husband-to-be—that's most important. It's fun shopping for a special gift. At the wedding you go out of your way to shake hands with the person you resent. The fact that you're having fun means a lot to your cousin. When it's over you have warm memories and good feelings about yourself.

THOUGHT FOR TODAY: A negative attitude is not just a state of mind, it can cause real harm.

If you have built castles in the air, your work need not be lost; that is where they should be. Now put foundations under them.

—Henry David Thoreau

I was always playing catch-up when I was drinking. My addiction took up almost all of my time, energy, and money. If I wasn't actually loaded, I was thinking about it, trying to get money for it, or trying to get straightened out.

Once I got sober, everything changed. I felt so much better. I became physically and emotionally capable of getting out in the world and enjoying myself. For the first time in years I had ambitions and dreams. I couldn't wait to rebuild my life.

Thankfully, a friend helped me keep my priorities in order during those early days of recovery. "Before you get carried away, don't forget that the structure of your new life is likely to be weak unless it's anchored to a solid foundation. The building process includes finding out who you really are, learning how to better interact with others, and getting into the habit of applying spiritual solutions to life's problems.

"Staying clean and sober, no matter what—that has to come first. You've probably learned the hard way that you can't achieve that on your own, so the most vital part of the foundation will be your relationship with God."

THOUGHT FOR TODAY: Your number one priority is staying clean and sober.

June 21

I do not know how the great loving Father will bring out light at last, but He knows and He will do it.

—David Livingstone

Some of us have undergone dramatic personality and behavioral changes that are often difficult to explain. When we're asked, "What happened? How did you do it?" the only thing we're able to say with certainty is, "*We didn't* do it—and that's the point."

After reflection, we realize we've had a spiritual awakening—a profound alteration of consciousness during which we became aware of God's power in our lives. By tapping into this inner resource of power, we brought about changes that seldom could have been accomplished even by years of self-discipline.

Spiritual awakenings sometimes come in sudden, dramatic realizations and awarenesses. A parent in paralyzing depression because of a child's tragic death finds the ability to face life again with the help of God. A person who is addicted to the point of seeming hopelessness finds that with God's power he can begin recovery; previously, without God's help, such an action had been absolutely impossible.

Most often, spiritual awakenings occur gradually. One's outlook and reaction to life evolves over a period of weeks, months, or years. In fact, a person may not even realize the degree of positive change that has taken place until it is pointed out by others.

THOUGHT FOR TODAY: The power of God can do for us what we cannot do for ourselves.

Perfect courage means doing unwitnessed what we would be capable of with the world looking on.
—Duc de La Rochefoucauld

For years I attributed my low self-worth to the unfair actions of other people. I've since discovered that my self-esteem tends to rise or fall in direct relation to the way *I* behave and think.

For example, I used to feel like a fraud because my behavior was in fact fraudulent. Naturally, I wanted to be well liked. So when the world was watching I would be careful, considerate, and well behaved. But when I was alone the mask came off. I didn't behave toward my family anywhere near the way I wanted others to *think* I did.

Stark honesty finally helped me realize how my two-faced behavior was undermining my feelings about myself. Deep down, I hated myself for my hypocritical behavior. It was time for me to start behaving differently. This would take courage and discipline, I was told. I was willing to try, and as a result I gradually learned to be consistent and regained my self-respect.

Today I try to do things because they are right. If, in the process, I gain the approval of others, well and good. The higher goal, though, is to gain approval from myself.

THOUGHT FOR TODAY: Masks can suffocate.

June 23

Peace of mind is that mental condition in which you have accepted the worst.

—Lin Yutang

When *acceptance* was first suggested as a solution to seemingly insurmountable problems, my immediate thought was, "That's easy for *you* to say!" But as time went by I discovered that acceptance can be practiced by anyone in any situation. Its rewards are not reserved solely for "spiritually experienced" people.

Today the goal is to accept circumstances and situations as they are, rather than as we wish them to be. When we "go with the flow" instead of trying to dodge adversity or bulldoze our way through it, the quality of our lives improves greatly.

First and foremost, acceptance brings release from our problems. Peace of mind follows, in contrast to the frustration and anxiety we had known before. Once calm, we are better able to listen to God and take action on His forthcoming guidance.

We have learned that the practice of acceptance need not be limited to serious eventualities such as illness. It can be practiced to great advantage on life's relatively minor misfortunes, offering a simple and effective remedy for the discomforts and aggravations we all face day-to-day.

THOUGHT FOR TODAY: Acceptance leads to peace of mind.

Fear of life in one form or another is the great thing to exorcise.

—William James

Experience has shown us again and again that our fears are almost always groundless—often to the point of total illusion. Yet that doesn't stop us from reacting fearfully each time the same situation or set of circumstances presents itself. Why haven't we been able to put this pervasive and corrosive emotion in its place?

It's probably because we tend to go around fearing or denying our feelings, instead of confronting and walking through them. Some of us have used drugs or alcohol to give ourselves false courage. We may depend on other people to run interference or be our "bodyguards." We sometimes disguise our fear with other emotions, such as anger or jealousy. Or we simply may not do anything and suffer in silence.

How can we better deal with our fears? Certainly we can reevaluate the situation; if we're willing to look at something from a new perspective, we'll often find it's not as threatening as it first appeared. Sometimes we can do this by asking ourselves, "What's the worst thing that can happen?"—or by talking to another person. The most effective way, we have found, is to reaffirm our belief and trust in God, and to ask for His help in replacing our fears with faith.

THOUGHT FOR TODAY: Our fears are almost always illusions.

June 25

Let me tell thee, time is a very precious gift of God; so precious that it's only given to us moment by moment.
—Amelia Barr

We often hear how important it is to "live in the now." We're told, and it's hard to disagree, that projection forward or backward causes us unnecessary worry and fear. When we are successful at remaining in the present, on the other hand, we benefit greatly.

By learning to live in the now, we first of all can truly appreciate the actuality of the moment. Because we're not just partially there—with our thoughts in yesterday or tomorrow—we're able to maximize our enjoyment of time spent with friends, in various activities, or simply relaxing.

When we're in the now and really paying attention, it's certainly a lot easier to remember what happened. This may not seem like much, but the advantages can be numerous. For one thing, our ability to retain information is enhanced; we can actually become better listeners. We're able to be a better friend by giving someone we care about a most valuable gift—our undivided attention. Living in the now also greatly increases our concentration, enabling us to improve our skills and do a better job in any number of areas.

All in all, life itself is more satisfying. *Now* we can do something about the present moment—or simply enjoy it to the fullest because we're *there*.

THOUGHT FOR TODAY: Live in the now.

It is the around-the-corner brand of hope that prompts people to action, while the distant hope acts as an opiate.
—Eric Hoffer

In the last few weeks of my drinking, I was convinced that I would never be able to quit and would likely die drunk. This belief had been reinforced during my most recent hospital stay, when a doctor had refused to treat me because I was "a loser."

Shortly after my release, a friend set up a meeting with someone he thought might be able to help me. I knew it would be a waste of time, but I agreed anyway.

That evening the man came to my house. He told me with surprising candor that just three years earlier he had been exactly where I was. "I had been in and out of hospitals, and I was about to lose my job and my home. And the thing was, the worse it got, the more impossible it was to quit."

He talked to me for several hours. In describing himself and his feelings, he described me. He seemed to know exactly how *I* felt—the loneliness, the desperation, the hopelessness.

What was even more astonishing about that evening, however, was the support and encouragement that was given to me. The man had been exactly where I was, yet he had gotten sober! For the first time in as long as I could remember, I had a glimmer of hope.

THOUGHT FOR TODAY: Hopelessness is more often a state of mind than a reality.

June 27

God is more truly imagined than expressed and He exists more truly than is imagined.

—St. Augustine

Throughout the ages, people have tried to conceptualize God. Musicians have attempted to capture His spirit in hymns and symphonies. Artists have portrayed the form of God in paintings and sculpture. Writers have created countless poems and stories in efforts to affirm His existence.

Certainly there is no harm in trying to express God in material terms. For many people, artful representations are necessary adjuncts to belief and faith. But more important than our ability to conceptualize God, we find, is knowing and experiencing the joyous realities of His presence and works in our lives.

Since coming to rely on God's power, we have discovered that He exists more truly than we could ever have imagined. This is evidenced by the miraculous ways in which our lives have been transformed.

We are free from addiction, worry, and fear. As a result, we are free to do things and experience life in ways that were previously impossible. Because of God's guidance, our lives have taken on new purpose and meaning. We are able to continue changing, and to help others do so. We understand what love is; because of God's love, we have learned to love ourselves and others.

THOUGHT FOR TODAY: Remember the joyous realities of God's presence and works in our lives.

And we ask not any soul to perform beyond its scope.
                                    —Koran, Sūrah 23

At times it seems that everybody is letting us down. We give our all to encourage and support our children, yet they continue to disappoint us. We enter a relationship with high hopes that a partner will share our desires and aspirations, but it turns out he or she wants something completely different. We feel betrayed. We haven't gotten so much as a pat on the back for the overtime we put in at work, and we feel taken for granted.

In each of these cases, clearly, we've become the victims of our own fixed expectations. We've written and choreographed an operetta with the fanciful idea that everyone will sing, dance, or otherwise perform exactly as we expect them to.

Obviously this is not the way of the world; only rarely will someone's actions match our expectations. People have the right to their *own* ideas and goals, to achieve their *own* successes and learn from their *own* mistakes.

It's time to stop setting ourselves up for disappointment. It's time to approach our relationships—indeed, life itself—without delusive expectations. It's time to simply let things happen the way they're supposed to, and stay out of the results.

THOUGHT FOR TODAY: It may be my script, but I'm not the director and it's certainly not my theater.

June 29

Bad temper is its own scourge.

—Charles Buxton

"When you get angry, you're the one who suffers," we're often told. "There's no place in your life for even so-called justifiable anger."

We may agree philosophically with this idea, and even pay it lip service. Deep down, however, we believe that in certain situations anger is the *only* appropriate response.

The day comes when we are confronted by one of these exceptions. We have been victims of a terrible injustice and are gravely offended. We seize the opportunity to erupt uncontrollably, causing a dramatic scene. We secretly relish not only our ability to vent our rage, but also the fact that we've disproven the theory. "Who says there's no such thing as justifiable anger?" we think with self-satisfaction.

But then time passes, perhaps only a short time. We begin to regret our behavior. We rehash the event over and over, each time feeling more embarrassment, guilt, and remorse. Before long we can't even sleep—we're sick because of what we've done.

Once again we've had to learn something the hard way—in this case the vital lesson that uncontrolled anger is an inappropriate response under any circumstance. It's simply not worth the suffering it causes us and those around us.

THOUGHT FOR TODAY: Anger is not a solution.

Life is a series of surprises. We do not guess today the mood, the pleasure, the power of tomorrow, when we are building up our being.

—Ralph Waldo Emerson

Very soon after we stop drinking or using, we begin to live again. The haunting memories of the past are stored for future reference as they are gradually augmented by uplifting new ones.

A friend told me about one of her first sober memories. While swimming in the ocean one day, she was surprised to see that she was coming very close to a pelican. When she got to within six feet, the bird tried to fly away, but could not. "It was all tangled up with fishing line," my friend said. "There was a hook in its beak, another one in its foot, and one in its wing."

She managed to maneuver the pelican to shore. With the help of others she captured the bird and extracted the hooks. "Then we set it free," she said. "I watched it soar, then barely skim the water, the way pelicans do."

"You must have felt great after that," I said.

"I did," she replied. "I really identified with that bird, with its newfound freedom. I had just been freed, too.

"Besides that," she added, "if I had been out there drunk, as I often was, I wouldn't even have noticed the pelican."

THOUGHT FOR TODAY: Today's sober joys will be tomorrow's joyful memories.

July 1

Even a thought, even a possibility can shatter us and transform us.

—Nietzsche

There were times in our old lives when, just for an instant, we could see ourselves and our circumstances in merciless reality. Such brief moments of clarity were startling and often extremely painful. We tried our best to quickly put them out of our minds, because we knew with dismal certainty that we couldn't change the way things were.

When we have such flashes of insight today, we usually welcome them, even though what we see can be upsetting. We try to recognize these illuminating experiences as major opportunities for increased self-awareness—as potent catalysts that can help bring about necessary changes in our lives.

To be sure, we're not always willing to follow through. However, most of the time after such moments of clarity, we do have the desire to take action. For we know from experience that our efforts will almost always result in marked growth.

When we are offered special awarenesses these days, we know how to bridge the gap between insight and actual change. We've learned what steps and procedures work when attitudes, behavior patterns, or situations in our lives require modification. We've been given tools for living and we know how to use them.

THOUGHT FOR TODAY: Action bridges the gap between a moment of clarity and actual change.

No viper so little, but hath its venom.

—Thomas Fuller

When our relationships haven't been as harmonious as we'd like them to be, and the people we are close to have seemed somewhat guarded, a certain amount of tension is obvious.

There are, of course, many reasons for tension in relationships. A common, yet frequently overlooked one is the use of sarcasm and teasing. Could it be that we've fallen into the habit of expressing ourselves in these ways—with the misguided idea that we're "just kidding around"?

The point is, there's no such thing as innocent sarcasm—any more than there is harmless teasing. When we poke fun at someone, we may feel that our motives are pure. But what do we actually do? Don't we in fact attack someone's weak spot or area of sensitivity? When we jokingly focus on a person's weight, hairline, or personality trait, aren't we trying to hurt him or her in some way—albeit a very small way?

This being the case, it might be a good idea to think about what took place when *we* were the victims of such actions. Actually, two injuries occurred. We were hurt, but probably didn't say anything. And the relationship was adversely affected. The next time we're tempted to be sarcastic or teasing, this awareness could change our minds.

THOUGHT FOR TODAY: The word *sarcasm* comes from the Greek word meaning "to tear flesh."

July 3

Pride is to character like the attic to the house—the highest part, and generally the most empty.

—John Gay

At the start of my recovery, I was told that if I wanted my life to truly change—and not just on the surface—I would have to search out the character flaws that caused my destructive behavior and, moreover, become willing to have those flaws removed. But I didn't really understand what was meant by "character flaws."

I was advised to consider a widely used list of major human defects—the so-called Seven Deadly Sins of pride, greed, lust, anger, gluttony, envy, and sloth. I was told that it would be helpful to concentrate first on pride, since that would be the primary obstacle to true progress for me.

For some time I found it difficult to see what pride really was and how it was manifesting itself in my life. I came to see, however, that for me pride is synonymous with dedication to selfishness, self-reliance, and self-centeredness—in other words, self in all its dimensions.

Consequently, when I am filled with pride, reliance upon my Higher Power is out of the question—and as a result, the quality of my life deteriorates.

THOUGHT FOR TODAY: Pride is a roadblock on the path to God.

Freedom is more precious than any gifts for which you may be tempted to give it up.

—Baltasar Gracián

It's easy to be inspired by historical accounts of nations and people fighting for their freedom. But what about our own personal freedom? How often do we even think about it? Probably hardly ever, because most of us tend to be complacent about our personal freedom.

The danger, as so many have learned, is that it's all too easy to lose what we take for granted.

We can lose our freedom all at once, simply by reverting to patterns that previously had enslaved us. We can jeopardize our freedom by making choices involving trade-offs—accepting a job offering more money and prestige, for example, but requiring us to give up cherished principles and career goals. Or, by our inaction, a more subtle erosion of our freedom can take place—if we remain in a relationship, for example, because it offers many "advantages"—even though it requires us to compromise our values and individuality.

Personal freedom in the final analysis is our individual responsibility, for it depends primarily on our choices and actions. If we are self-honest, especially concerning motives, if we seek God's guidance, and if we then courageously strive to make the right choices and take the right actions, it's likely we will not only preserve but also strengthen our personal freedom.

THOUGHT FOR TODAY: Choose to be free.

July 5

Thou hast touched me and I have been transformed into thy peace.

—St. Augustine

When we are distressed and have difficulty concentrating or relaxing, we know we can turn to God for relief. Even when we feel incapable of prayer, we can try to be still, allowing our minds and bodies to rest in the comforting presence of God. We can close our eyes and feel God's peace flowing through us, replacing our inner discord with harmony.

As we allow God's peace to fill our minds and hearts, anxiety and overblown cares leave us. God's peace is pure and vibrant, disallowing ideas and concerns not in accord with His perfection.

A feeling of calm begins to pervade our whole being when we turn to God. With this renewing flow comes a healing of emotions, mind, and body. We are filled with tranquil thoughts, which guide us in ways of working and living harmoniously with others.

When we turn to God in these ways and He brings comfort and reassurance, we are once again reminded that He has the power to bring peace and harmony to all persons and situations.

THOUGHT FOR TODAY: God's peace can restore me, replacing inner discord with harmony.

We are all but stewards of what we falsely call our own; yet avarice is so insatiable that it is not in the power of abundance to content it.

—Seneca

Only now, in retrospect, do we fully realize the extent to which greed ruled our lives. We're not surprised that this character defect is among the Seven Deadly Sins, for our avarice knew no bounds. We relentlessly sought not only money and possessions, but also ever-increasing amounts of prestige, attention, and approval.

We also see clearly that our greed was but the surface manifestation of our underlying problem—a deep void within us caused by insecurity, fear, and a sense of purposelessness.

There came a time of revelation when we *knew* that nothing material could ever fill the "hole in our gut." For we discovered that our lifelong sense of bankruptcy was of a spiritual nature. Soon thereafter, we made a decision to turn our lives over to the care of God.

We embarked on a spiritual journey, and along the way have been given riches that we could never find or accumulate on our own—a sense of usefulness and belonging, serenity, and genuine happiness. Today we know that we can best remain spiritually fulfilled through service to God—and we can best serve Him by giving of ourselves to others.

THOUGHT FOR TODAY: Greed is the surface manifestation of an inner spiritual void.

July 7

Our worth is determined by the good deeds we do, rather than by the fine emotions we feel.

—Elias Magoon

I considered myself a compassionate and sympathetic person. My heart went out to the downtrodden and those in need; I was always on the side of the underdog.

Looking back, I see that I took a great deal of pride in that character trait, even though I rarely lifted a finger to help anyone but myself. The empty feelings of empathy allowed me to rationalize on occasion that I was a good-natured, caring person. Moreover, my self-deception convinced me that since I had this one virtue, I must have had many.

When I began my new life and gradually became willing to take an honest look at myself, this rationalization was one of the first to fall away. I had to admit that my actual behavior and attitudes belied my pumped up self-image. In reality I was intolerant, unkind, and, more than anything, self-centered.

I realize now that sympathy and compassion must carry responsibility with them if they are to have any real meaning. When I am moved with compassion these days, I make an effort to reach out and put my feelings into action.

THOUGHT FOR TODAY: True sympathy and compassion include action.

It is well to give when asked, but it is better to give unasked, through understanding.

—Kahlil Gibran

To one degree or another we are all self-obsessed at the beginning of our new life. One of the best ways to get out of ourselves and become less self-centered, we're told, is by helping others. We're also taught that we need not wait for any certain "level" of development before doing this. It's never too early; actually, the sooner the better.

Some people think that to "be of service" one needs to take actions that are obvious and even dramatic. This isn't the case at all. Often, in fact, the most unobtrusive acts can be the most helpful and meaningful.

We feel better about ourselves when we are serving others, there's no question about that. Our lives take on greater purpose and meaning. At the same time our faith deepens because of our strengthened partnership with God.

And that for us is really the main point. From our own experience we have learned that God works through people. That is how He came into our lives. Through service we can help bring Him into the lives of others.

THOUGHT FOR TODAY: Service to others is a sure-fire remedy for self-absorption.

July 9

The fox condemns the trap, not himself.

—William Blake

There are traps in daily living; that's the way the world is. People sometimes take their problems out on us, blame us for their mistakes, or try to take advantage of us. There are communication breakdowns; we do something based on incomplete instructions, and it turns out wrong.

Before I began my recovery I was so filled with guilt and lacking in self-esteem that I tended automatically to assume responsibility for many of the traps in my life. I blamed myself for mishaps that had nothing to do with me or my abilities. I was willing to be just about everybody's scapegoat.

I remember how good it felt the first time I stood up for myself in sobriety. To actually confront a false accusation was so exhilarating that I decided to write about the experience and then share my thoughts with a spiritual adviser. By taking those actions, I was able to see how extensive my blame taking had been, how much I had been damaged, and what I needed to do to break the pattern once and for all.

When things go wrong these days, when life occasionally throws a punch in my direction, I no longer feel the need to apologize for "being in the way" of the fist. Most of the time, in fact, I'm able to dodge the blow and continue on with the business of living.

THOUGHT FOR TODAY: We can remain free of self-reproach even when we're "trapped."

There is no vulture like despair.

—George Granville

Despite the joys and riches of our new lives, practically all of us reexperience feelings of despair. These feelings may be our reaction to actual tragedies. More often, however, we have a sense of not being able to cope with all the things that demand our attention. No matter what the cause when we are in despair, we feel hopelessness and futility.

One of the greatest rewards of our spiritual awakening is that we learn enduring lessons that can be applied and reapplied. In the case of despair, haven't we learned that our painful feelings only *seem* like they will last forever, that our problems only *appear* to be unsolvable? If we feel that everything is helpless and hopeless, isn't it true that our minds have distorted reality?

When we are filled with despair, let us remind ourselves that things always work out (sometimes in unexpected ways) when we unreservedly give up and ask God for help. At that point our feelings of futility are transformed—we surrender and allow ourselves to be rejuvenated by God's power and grace.

THOUGHT FOR TODAY: Despair is often a distorted reflection of reality.

July 11

Live near to God, and so all things will appear to you little in comparison with eternal realities.

—R. M. M'Cheyne

Am I too busy to take fifteen minutes from my day to communicate with God? If my answer is yes, then I can't afford *not* to take the time—because that's when I probably need it most. I've learned that if I am not careful, a continually stressful schedule can cause me to feel separated from God. In time this hinders my spiritual growth.

What happens when I reorder my priorities and set aside time for prayer and meditation? Almost immediately I feel a sense of peace and calmness, knowing that God is with me and I no longer need to rely solely on my own resources.

Because I have opened myself to Him, I am far more likely to receive His guidance. It may not come during my actual period of meditation. But experience has taught me that it will come at some point—either in the form of a special inspiration that seemingly comes out of nowhere, or as an intuitive feeling deep within me.

When I take the time to communicate with God, I am refreshed and renewed. My day can begin anew, and it's likely that I'll be more successful at what I'm doing.

THOUGHT FOR TODAY: When you're too busy for prayer and meditation, that's probably when you need it most.

The greatest thing in the world is to know how to be one's own self.

—Michel Eyquem de Montaigne

The scenario is a familiar one. An employer, friend, mate, or family member is going through a rough time. The person is behaving erratically and is extremely difficult to get along with. He (or she) may be taking his troubles out on us, being unjust, demanding, or simply hurtful. Our tendency has been to take such behavior personally—to get into the act by becoming upset and angry, or fighting back.

It's almost impossible *not* to be affected when people we're close to go off the deep end. But that doesn't mean we have to jump off right behind them. We do ourselves a great disservice when we allow others to color our attitude and ruin our day.

These are the times when we must do whatever it takes to maintain our serenity, security, and happiness. We've gone to great lengths to gain personal freedom, and these days we think twice before letting someone else interfere with it even temporarily. Moreover, whenever we permit another person's difficulties to compromise our own values and objectives, we lose whatever chance we may have to be understanding, encouraging, and helpful.

THOUGHT FOR TODAY: The behavior of others need not dictate our unhappiness or discomfort.

July 13

The shortest and surest way to live with honor in the world is to be in reality what we would appear to be.

—Socrates

Once in a while we're given the opportunity to see ourselves as we used to be. We're at a social gathering, say, and someone there is going to great lengths to make everyone notice and like him.

At first we're put off by his behavior, but soon we watch with fascination. It's like viewing a video playback of our own phoniness in the past. We, too, worked hard at presenting an image that we thought would attract others and win approval. It was important to appear charming, on top of things, enviable.

As we watch, several things occur to us. We realize how much time and energy we used to put into presenting an image—and how sadly misdirected it all was. We see how much better off we are now that we're putting our efforts into a far worthier goal: becoming in reality the person we once pretended to be, by actually acquiring the character traits we felt others would admire.

We are also reminded that we didn't make the transition automatically. It has taken willingness, self-honesty, self-awareness, and action.

THOUGHT FOR TODAY: The person you wanted to be has always been within you.

Repetition is reality, and it is the seriousness of life.
—Sören Kierkegaard

No matter how convinced we are that spirituality works, we all occasionally try again to do things "our way." The results are always the same. We wonder then how we could have forgotten that a life run on self-will rather than God's will makes for a bumpy, uncomfortable ride.

When we temporarily revert to our old ways, we shouldn't be too hard on ourselves. After all, learning and applying spiritual principles isn't like riding a bike; just because we've been initially successful doesn't mean we'll automatically remember how to do it or, for that matter, *why* we should do it.

To remain spiritually fit and to offset our capricious old ideas, we need to return regularly and often to the "well." We can do this by maintaining contact with spiritually aware people, and by prayer and meditation. We can also frequently remind ourselves that spirituality provides us a way to live comfortably and serenely.

If we take these actions, can we be guaranteed immediate progress? Not necessarily. However, we will most definitely make progress over time. We know from experience the advantages of learning and then relearning spiritual principles. The better we know and understand them, the more effectively we can apply them, and the better the quality of our lives.

THOUGHT FOR TODAY: Spiritual fitness can be enhanced by repetition, not by rhetoric; by practice, not by preaching.

July 15

Worry is a form of fear, and all forms of fear produce fatigue. A man who has learned not to feel fear will find the fatigue of daily life enormously diminished.
— Bertrand Russell

I'm sick and tired of worrying about things that don't really matter.

I'm sick and tired of having unreasonable expectations of myself.

I'm sick and tired of worrying about things over which I have no control.

I'm sick and tired of worrying about what other people are thinking about me.

I'm sick and tired of taking my emotional temperature.

I'm sick and tired of using my energy foolishly by regretting what happened yesterday and worrying about what might happen tomorrow.

I'm sick and tired of comparing my insides to other people's outsides.

I'm sick and tired of being so hard on myself.

I'm sick and tired of waiting until the last minute, and causing myself problems by putting things off.

I'm sick and tired of feeling sorry for myself.

I'm sick and tired of living in the problem instead of the solution.

I'm sick and tired of being sick and tired.

THOUGHT FOR TODAY: FEAR = False Evidence Appearing Real.

You may find the worst enemy or best friend within yourself.
　　　　　　　　　　　　　　　　—English proverb

Because of our low self-esteem, we unwittingly made choices that placed us in physical or emotional jeopardy. We spent time with "lower companions," or took foolish risks. Beyond such real hazards, it seemed that the world was booby-trapped with pitfalls and dangers of every kind, that everyone and everything was out to get us. As it turned out, the greatest dangers we faced were from ourselves.

For a long time we lacked the self-honesty to admit what we were doing, and the self-awareness to understand why we were doing it. Gradually, however, we learned that we could make self-fulfilling rather than self-destructive choices. We realized that we could be our own best friend rather than our own worst enemy.

Today, as a result, we take actions to enhance our physical and emotional well-being, rather than allowing ourselves to become run-down to the point of collapse. Because we care enough about ourselves, we avoid potentially damaging situations and relationships—rather than seeking them out. In every possible way, in thoughts as well as actions, we are respectful rather than contemptuous of ourselves.

THOUGHT FOR TODAY: Be kind to yourself.

July 17

Self-reverence, self-knowledge, self-control; these three alone lead life to sovereign power.

—Alfred Tennyson

"I just walked away from a twenty-year relationship and I'm really confused about how I feel," a newly sober friend confided. "I'm proud for having the guts to do what's necessary, but I feel like crying my eyes out."

She explained that she and her friend had been sorority sisters, and had stayed close through their subsequent marriages and child-raising years. "We drank together through it all. Then when I got sober, the relationship began to deteriorate. I still care about her, but it's just not the same. Today I decided I can't see her anymore, not for a while."

At first my friend's sobriety wasn't taken seriously. But soon her longtime friend began making antagonistic remarks about her new life. "She insisted that I couldn't be an alcoholic, and kept trying to get me to drink with her. She started baiting me, saying things like, 'What's all this spiritual garbage?' "

I told my friend that she had made an important and courageous decision by putting her recovery first, and that the relationship might even be restored one day. "That's true," she agreed. "It would be a terrible mistake to let anything get in the way of my sobriety. But knowing that doesn't make it hurt any the less right now."

THOUGHT FOR TODAY: Recovery begins with a willingness to do whatever it takes.

I always say to myself, what is the most important thing we can think about at this extraordinary moment.

—R. Buckminster Fuller

There are times when life seems much more fulfilling and exciting than usual. Conversations with other people are interesting, almost without exception. We are stimulated by sights, sounds, and events that at other times have seemed completely mundane.

The difference is not in the interactions or occurrences, but in the level of our enthusiasm. When we are enthusiastic, our minds are unclouded and our vision is clearly focused. We are better able to absorb, understand, and appreciate what is going on around us. There is always something new to explore and enjoy.

At home or at work, our enthusiasm brings about deeper appreciation for family members and friends. We listen to their ideas and opinions in an entirely different way.

When we are enthusiastic, we express positive energy that is often contagious. Our enthusiasm can not only transform ordinary goings-on into richly rewarding experiences, but can also bring about a similar attitude in those around us.

If we can remain enthusiastic today, we will be alert and open to pleasures we might otherwise miss. As we respond enthusiastically to this day, so will we derive joy and satisfaction as it unfolds.

THOUGHT FOR TODAY: When I am enthusiastic there is always something new to explore and enjoy.

July 19

Self-sacrifice enables us to sacrifice other people without blushing.
—George Bernard Shaw

We all know people who are self-styled martyrs. Most of them are convinced that they would be happier, more successful, indeed, much better off in *all* ways, if that certain person hadn't mistreated them, or if they hadn't become a "victim of circumstances."

What are some of the consequences when we choose to blame others for the conditions of our lives? First and foremost, we absolve ourselves of responsibility for our problems and state of mind. In effect, we give ourselves permission not to seek solutions, not to act—not to change. The end result is that we remain stuck in the situation.

There is no plus side to martyrdom. It's a bumpy and punishing trip all the way. However, if we become willing to get on with the business of living, there are ways to break out of this paralyzing form of self-centeredness.

Rather than focusing on ourselves as victims, we can try to focus on solutions. One day at a time, we can strive to accept what has happened—no matter how we feel about it. Most important, we can ask a loving God to show us the way as we begin to take responsibility for our lives.

THOUGHT FOR TODAY: Martyrs are victimized not so much by others as by themselves.

What loneliness is more lonely than distrust?

—George Eliot

In my old life I refused to trust anyone. It was the only way I knew how to live. When I saw people trusting one another, my immediate thought was how foolish they were. Since I couldn't be trusted, I reasoned, nobody else could be.

I've come to realize that my attitude stemmed in large measure from my own negative feelings about myself. I was totally dishonest in the way I presented myself to others—rarely did I allow anyone to see me as I actually was. My lack of trust therefore had very little to do with the untrustworthiness of others—and everything to do with my fears that I would be "found out."

When my life turned around, among the first essentials was learning to trust myself, others, and God. It was necessary for me to become honest about who I really was, and to be willing to put that person on the line. I had to gradually risk being vulnerable.

It took time, but I slowly developed confidence and trust in the integrity of others. The more trustworthy I became in my activities and relationships, the more trusting I became of my fellows.

THOUGHT FOR TODAY: The more trustworthy you are, the more trusting of others you will become.

July 21

The beginning of love is to let those we love be perfectly themselves, and not to twist them to fit our own image. Otherwise we love only the reflection of ourselves we find in them.

—Thomas Merton

God's love for us is not contingent on the degree to which we please or displease Him or, for that matter, on any set of standards. God loves us unconditionally.

Now that we have come to know this, we aspire to love others in the same way. While we realize that God alone is capable of perfectly unconditional love, we believe it is His will that we strive for progress in that direction.

We have learned that the first step is a willingness to accept others as they are. It is only then that we can begin to love them as they are, without self-seeking motives. What this means in practical terms is trying to be loving toward our families and friends regardless of their behavior, attitudes, or opinions.

This is an unquestionably lofty and difficult objective, yet it becomes increasingly attainable as we acquire greater humility. We decrease the need to tie strings to our love as we become less self-involved. We heighten our ability to love others unconditionally as we grow spiritually and become more secure within ourselves.

THOUGHT FOR TODAY: The first step toward unconditional love is accepting others as they are.

Experience is a hard teacher. She gives the test first and the lessons afterward.

—Anonymous

No one would argue that the best way to learn anything is through personal experience. But these days we're able to learn in other ways as well. We learn from other people, because we've finally become willing to open our minds and listen to them. And we learn from our own common sense and intuition.

In the past many of us were poor students no matter what the source of the lesson. We resisted listening to reason, sometimes to the point of recalcitrance. When we were warned against taking a certain path, we rebelliously veered in that direction. Our egos told us that we had all the answers—or, if we didn't, we could certainly find them without outside help.

What changed for us? The most important thing was that we became aware of our limitations. We grew tired of being our own biggest stumbling blocks—of having to learn everything the hard way. By gradually becoming open-minded and trusting of others, we were able to learn from them without having to repeat their mistakes—or make our own.

This is not to say that we've stopped learning from our own experiences; but now that we're teachable, we can assimilate our lessons more quickly and effectively.

THOUGHT FOR TODAY: By benefiting from the experiences of others, you can learn lessons without needless suffering.

July 23

Somebody's boring me . . . I think it's me.

—Dylan Thomas

In the second year of my sobriety I went through a period of profound boredom. It seemed that nothing new was happening at work, at home, or in any other area of my life. A sense of disillusionment nibbled away at me. I began to wonder spiritlessly what I had to look forward to.

One night during that time, I went to a movie by myself. Images flashed by as I stared at the screen, but nothing registered. I was thinking how boring life had become, and that it had never been like that before.

From childhood, in fact, just the opposite had been true. I had lived a roller coaster existence. I would go straight up and then come crashing downward—again and again and again. Everything had been high drama, and most of it had been of my own making.

As I sat there in the darkness, I suddenly realized that for quite some time, my life had actually been on an even keel. If anything was missing, it was the turmoil and the constant ups and downs. It dawned on me that I wasn't experiencing boredom at all, but something that I had longed for all my life—*serenity*. It was actually in my grasp, and to this day it remains within reach.

THOUGHT FOR TODAY: What appears at first to be boredom may be the harbinger of serenity.

The real voyage of discovery consists not in seeking new landscapes, but in having new eyes.

—Marcel Proust

Sometimes, extraordinarily, we undergo a spiritual experience. A sequence of events, more often than not, serves to bring about inexplicable and even mysterious changes within us. From that point on, we see things differently—frequently in an entirely new light.

The world around us—our jobs, relationships, possessions—may be exactly the same as before. But because of our spiritual experience, we have been given the opportunity and the insight to discover things about ourselves and our lives that we had not been able to see before.

We may, for example, gain a new understanding and compassion for parents with whom we've never really gotten along. In the process, we realize how much we actually love them. Perhaps we become sharply aware for the first time that it's necessary to change careers. Or revelations about ourselves may open the door to unexpected new personal freedoms.

When we look back at these exceptional transformations, we can see that while we had nothing to do with bringing them about, the opportunity would have passed us by had we not been open-minded, willing, and receptive.

THOUGHT FOR TODAY: Today and every day, open your mind and heart as well as your eyes.

July 25

No one can make you feel inferior without your consent.
                                        —Eleanor Roosevelt

Self-awareness has become one of our most valued character assets. Today we know where we stand—not only with ourselves, but in the world.

This was not always the case. In the past our awareness of self had an obsessive quality; it manifested itself in negative ways, such as painful self-consciousness and a gnawing sense of being "different." Because we were uncomfortable when we met new people, for example, we were quite willing to change our appearances, mannerisms, and opinions in order to blend in. Some of us were willing to change everything about ourselves.

Eventually, thank God, we grew tired of not having identities of our own. We made honest self-appraisals and discovered that, along with the flaws, there actually were things we liked about ourselves. By focusing on those good qualities, we found the courage to start developing our own styles.

Little by little we began to accept our true selves. We became less afraid to express our opinions, even if they were controversial or unpopular. We realized that we didn't have to act like chameleons anymore—most people accept us just the way we are. And we feel better about ourselves than we ever have.

THOUGHT FOR TODAY: By being true to yourself, you're true to others.

Dios tarda pero no olvida. God delays but doesn't forget.
—Spanish proverb

At times God seems remote and incomprehensible. We experience frustration in establishing conscious contact with Him. Even though we know this can happen occasionally, our knowledge doesn't keep us from growing impatient or even irritated with ourselves and God. The longer such disquieting episodes go on, the more spiritless and alone we feel.

The best way to get through these periods, we have found, is by acting "as if." Despite what our minds have begun to tell us, we trust our hearts and continue praying for awareness of God's will. We continue to meditate, which is our way of remaining open to His response. Ultimately, we undergo a spiritual experience through which our conscious contact with God becomes restored.

There is no way of knowing or predicting how, where, or when this restoration will occur. It can take place during meditation—or, no less likely, while we're shopping in a supermarket. We have come to realize that we're not meant to know how, where, or when God will disclose Himself to us. Trust in God means not having to know.

THOUGHT FOR TODAY: When God seems remote, trust your heart rather than your mind.

The talkative listen to no one, for they are ever speaking. And the first evil that attends those who know not how to be silent is that they hear nothing.

—Plutarch

We've learned that open-mindedness is vital to our progress. We know that in order to absorb new ideas and to find new solutions, we have to be teachable and receptive. For many of us, however, a major obstacle to achieving open-mindedness is our lifelong habit of focusing on nothing but ourselves and our problems.

When we finally come into contact with people who seem to be knowledgeable and understanding, we can't resist dominating the conversation. Expounding endlessly on our troubles, we whine and complain—we talk, talk, talk. We rehash the same old self-centered and self-destructive ideas that have kept us miserable for so long. Needless to say, when we do this we deny ourselves the opportunity to learn from others and to receive new input.

Granted that it's a relief to finally open up after years of feeling misunderstood and alone. Indeed, it's necessary to do so in order to get help. But after a point we have to keep our mouths closed and our ears open—we have to shut up and listen.

THOUGHT FOR TODAY: Closing your mouth can lead to opening your mind.

How poor are they who have not patience! What wound did ever heal but by degrees?

—William Shakespeare

In the early days of recovery, the first urgent requirement is to become physically sober. We must become detoxified before we can even think about doing anything else.

Initially most of us sought help solely to stop drinking or using drugs or overeating. But when our bodies were free of chemicals and our minds became somewhat clear, we were told that our dependencies were but symptoms of our disease. To stay sober and recover in the broadest sense, we would have to patiently deal with the real problem—our living problem. We would have to reach deep within ourselves to uncover and excise the roots and causes of our addictions.

In my own case, it took me a while before I understood. I finally "got it" one night when I heard a young woman's grateful comments as she celebrated one year of sobriety.

"When a horse gets a deep cut and the scar tissue heals over it," she said, "the wound itself isn't really healed. You have to reopen the wound by peeling away that top layer of scar tissue. You have to keep doing that.

"That top layer is called proud flesh," she added. "You have to keep stripping it away until the wound heals from inside. And that's what recovery has been for me—an inside job."

THOUGHT FOR TODAY: Getting sober or clean is part of it; learning to live is all of it.

July 29

If I am faithful to the duties of the present, God will provide for the future.

—Gregory T. Bedell

It's hard to dispute the wisdom and value of living in the present moment. We know from experience that when we do, we're much more comfortable and serene. Yet as convinced as we are of the soundness of this concept, it's difficult for most of us to consistently stay in the now. It's not as if we can wake up one morning and say, "I've got it!" and then automatically practice the principle forever after.

That's why many of us begin each day by affirming our willingness to live in the present, and by making conscious decisions about the twenty-four hours ahead.

We resolve today to live in the now—to accept the responsibilities and rewards of each unfolding moment. We commit ourselves to "be there" mentally as well as physically. By concentrating on what's directly in front of us moment by moment, we can usually accomplish these goals successfully and consistently.

We approach the day in a state of surrender, placing our faith and trust in God. We are determined to do the best we can in the present moment. And we resolve to leave the results to God.

THOUGHT FOR TODAY: Make a conscious decision, right now, to live in the now.

Find the grain of truth in criticism—chew it and swallow it.
—D. Sutten

Nobody likes to be criticized; we all know that from experience. Some of us, though, find it impossible to accept even mild and well-intentioned suggestions. We become immediately angry and defensive without even thinking about the point being made. At the very least these episodes can be painful and embarrassing; at the worst they can destroy relationships.

One mistake we sometimes make is to focus on the "messenger" rather than the message. It's easy to become offended when we think, and possibly say, "How dare you criticize me, when your faults are so much worse than mine!" We may even be tempted to retaliate if we feel the other person is simply "out to get us."

Looking at criticism another way, we can only go so far in evaluating our own actions and attitudes. If we want to make continuing progress in our lives, we should at least become willing to hear people out.

Of course, that doesn't mean just because someone criticizes us we have to automatically agree. But if we find we disagree after rationally evaluating the remarks, we don't have to react defensively. By trying to be gracious and tactful to our critic, we can turn a potentially negative experience into a positive one.

THOUGHT FOR TODAY: Sometimes the only way we can see ourselves clearly is through the eyes of another.

July 31

The tragedy of life is not so much what men suffer, but rather what they miss.

—Thomas Carlyle

No one can avoid tragedies such as serious illness, separation, and the loss of a loved one. Each of us is greatly challenged from time to time; that is part of life. So too is the suffering we go through as the result of such tragedies.

Certainly we have no control over the occurrences themselves. To an extent we are also powerless over our reactions to them. There comes a time, however, when we can make choices.

Some people choose to continue suffering, literally repatterning their lives around the calamity. They become imprisoned by self-pity and grow accustomed to the pity of others. They may become reclusive and lose their vitality. The overall consequences can be as tragic as the original event.

The far better choice is to try to put the tragedy behind us, do what it takes to move forward, and get on with our lives. This is rarely easy to accomplish. But it definitely can be done if we're determined to regain our zest for living.

We need time to make the transitional steps from shock and grief to acceptance and renewal. We need the support of family and friends, as well as professionals in some cases. In any case, the choice and responsibility are ours—and so are the benefits.

THOUGHT FOR TODAY: Powerlessness does not include our ability to make choices.

God grant me the serenity to accept the things I cannot change, the courage to change the things I can, and the wisdom to know the difference.

—Reinhold Niebuhr

Used by millions of people throughout the world, the Serenity Prayer offers comfort, reassurance, and a lot more. Its popularity and effectiveness lie in the fact that it provides clear and simple spiritual solutions to any kind of living problem.

What is it we're really asking for when we use the Serenity Prayer? The first part of the prayer has to do with powerlessness and acceptance. We acknowledge our lack of power over people, places, and things—and we ask God to help us accept them as they are.

The second part of the prayer deals with willingness and courage. We indicate that we have the willingness to take responsibility and do our part—the "footwork." We ask God for the courage to take action in situations where our footwork is necessary.

In the last part of the prayer we express recognition that it's often difficult, on our own, to know which situations require acceptance and which require action. We ask God to guide us, to indicate His will for us, to make His wisdom known to us. Clearly, there's much more to the Serenity Prayer than we might have thought.

THOUGHT FOR TODAY: We can achieve serenity through acceptance, action, and the willingness to seek and do God's will.

August 2

It's what you learn after you know it all that counts.
—John Wooden

Like so many practicing alcoholics, when I was drinking nobody could tell me anything I didn't already know. I was an expert on every subject, from politics and sports to medicine and high finance. I never said, "I don't know." Even if I didn't understand the question, I would make up an answer.

As a teenager I pretended to have all the answers because I didn't want people to think I was stupid. Later on, I had "delusions of grandeur" and truly believed that I knew it all. Toward the end, I tried to act knowledgeable to hide my confusion.

Over time my motives changed, but my behavior remained essentially the same. Even when I was put into a mental institution because of my alcoholism, I had all the answers. I "treated" patients with a wide range of mental disorders. Looking back, it's a wonder they let me out.

I'm not like that anymore, thank God. What a relief not to have to maintain that image, pretending I'm knowledgeable in areas where I know little or nothing. Today I have the freedom to say, "I don't know." This, in turn, leads to other freedoms—open-mindedness and the motivation to learn, humility, and the freedom to seek answers elsewhere and to respect the knowledge and opinions of others.

THOUGHT FOR TODAY: Learning to say "I don't know" is a key to open-mindedness, growth, and knowledge.

Nothing astonishes men so much as common sense and plain dealing.

—Ralph Waldo Emerson

We've progressed beyond the point where we question the necessity for complete honesty in our lives. Self-honesty, we've learned, is vital to improving the way we feel about ourselves. It leads to self-awareness and, in turn, to the possibility of positive changes in our entire outlook. Honesty in our relationships and interactions with others is, of course, just as important.

Like everybody else, we're faced with the daily influences of the outside world. Because of our new instincts and priorities, however, we know what choice to make. Not only do we avoid the temptation to be dishonest by *commission*—taking something that doesn't belong to us—we also avoid dishonesty by *omission*. If we receive high praise for a job well done, for example, and no mention is made of an assistant's invaluable participation, we speak up rather than passively accept all the credit for ourselves.

Sometimes others find our actions surprising, or even "stupid." But regardless of peer or societal pressures, we insist on remaining unwaveringly honest in all our affairs. For us, compromise means regression and possible disaster.

THOUGHT FOR TODAY: For me, honesty isn't simply the best policy, it's the only policy.

August 4

If you want to be miserable, think about yourself, about what you want, what you like, what respect people ought to pay you, and what people think of you.

—Charles Kingsley

Looking back, many of us can see that we were "egomaniacs with inferiority complexes." As a result, we tended to think, act, and react in extremes. There was no middle ground of equality—we felt either "better than" or "less than."

In a sense we lived double lives. Though we ached on the inside, we often behaved in ways designed to convince others that we were better and more important than everyone else. As time went on, our disguises wore thin. We became terrified that our true identity of "worthlessness" would be revealed for all the world to see.

Today we realize that actions and thoughts motivated strictly by self-centeredness can bring us only misery. Our recovery from egomania depends on thinking about and doing what we can for others, rather than constantly worrying about what they can do for us.

When we think of everyone as equal, and act accordingly, we feel best about ourselves.

THOUGHT FOR TODAY: You are neither better nor worse, but equal.

God gives us the nuts, but He does not crack them.

—German proverb

When we enter the realm of spiritual thought and activity, we are presented with a cornucopia of concepts that promise to enhance our lives: the rewards of faith, the power of prayer and meditation in gaining knowledge of God's will, the value of trust in Him. As we excitedly explore these concepts, we find that they are actually tools that, when regularly applied, can bring us joy and freedom.

But occasionally some of us temporarily lose perspective. We're so impressed by the miracles that have already taken place in our lives, we expect them to keep happening without any effort on our part.

Perhaps at that point we pray for something we think we need—and don't get it. The first small doubts about our faith may begin to creep in. We may even start to experience the same sense of futility we so often felt in the past.

Soon we realize that we need to get back into action. We again understand that although God most assuredly provides the power and the opportunities, we must do the footwork. By our action—our works of faith—we not only demonstrate our willingness to Him, but also enjoy our spirituality more completely because we're fully involved.

THOUGHT FOR TODAY: We must work for the rewards of faith.

August 6

Quiet minds cannot be perplexed or frightened, but go on in fortune or misfortune at their own private pace, like a clock during a thunderstorm.

—Robert Louis Stevenson

Sometimes it seems that a committee of doomsayers has taken over my mind, filling it with negative thoughts that have no basis in reality. The longer I allow the committee to remain in session, the louder and more threatening it becomes—and the more tense and anxious I become.

Thankfully, I have a choice in the matter these days. I've already "switched stations" insofar as my life-style and attitudes are concerned, so it's become much easier to tune out fearful and undesirable thoughts.

More importantly, I am learning to quiet my mind. I do so not only for the immediate relief it brings, but in preparation for a longer-term benefit.

When I quiet my mind I become ready for God's guidance to be revealed to me. Through my trust in Him I achieve calmness even during times of great stress—even when those all around me are agitated. I achieve calmness, which is constructive of good in my life. I achieve calmness and in the process become once again grateful for God's power and grace.

THOUGHT FOR TODAY: Strive for a quiet mind.

I have never been able to conceive how any rational being could propose happiness to himself from the exercise of power over others.

—Thomas Jefferson

A manager's responsibilities can range from controlling employees and processes to meeting profit objectives. That's why good managers are highly valued and often well paid. But in addition to these individuals, there are those who assume management responsibilities for which they are neither valued nor paid.

There is the parent, for example, who constantly tries to run the lives of her adult children—their relationships, careers, and even their pregnancies. For most of us, though, managing may consist solely of frequent suggestions on how others should dress or spend their time.

In either case, we may have gotten into the habit of managing others without realizing it. Perhaps at one point we were forced into the role and haven't been able to let it go. Or we may unwittingly try to make ourselves look good through the behavior, appearance, or achievements of those around us.

What happens when we try to manage others? For one thing, we show a lack of respect for their rights as individuals. We also deprive them of the opportunity to learn from their own decisions and choices. In some cases, we can erode the dignity and self-respect of those we love the most.

THOUGHT FOR TODAY: When I try to manage others, I'm not in control but "out of control."

August 8

Beginnings are apt to be shadowy.

—Rachel Carson

During the first weeks of recovery, our lives are usually in such turmoil that we see the need to quickly set a course toward new objectives. Time passes, and to our delight things begin to get better. Although we realize we have a long way to go, we're pleased with our progress. Then suddenly, for various reasons—or no apparent reason—we relapse into drinking, drug use, or other dependency. We "slip."

Just because we've temporarily fallen short of our goals doesn't mean they're impossible to achieve. We're certainly not doomed to a prolonged relapse, nor do we need to feel guilty or ashamed.

Those of us who have made continuing progress in recovery have come to understand that we slipped for a reason. When we asked ourselves what went wrong, we discovered one or more probabilities: Our foundation was weak, our relapse resulted from a buildup of negative thinking, our motives for recovery were unsound, or maybe we simply weren't ready to stop.

When we got back on course we realized it was an ideal time to review our goals and perhaps plan a new strategy. We carefully examined our motives and priorities to see if they were sound and in order. We sought help. And we began again, one day at a time.

THOUGHT FOR TODAY: We can learn from a relapse.

Only man clogs his happiness with care, destroying what is with thoughts of what may be.

—John Dryden

We spend some days shuttling back and forth between the past and the future. There are revealing phrases that usually go along with our mental time-travel. Don't we often find ourselves saying we *should've, would've,* or *could've* done something else? Haven't we frequently told ourselves that we *ought to, need to,* or *have to* do one thing or another?

We all fall into this trap, with the unfortunate result of ruining our ability to use and enjoy the present moment. We've just moved into our hard-earned first house, for example. Instead of savoring the moment, we manage to take all the joy out of it by thinking it *would've* been better to buy a condo. Or we've just reached our vacation destination and are already miserable because we're telling ourselves we *should've* gone somewhere else.

Even in less significant circumstances, we often concentrate on what we *have to, need to,* or *should* do. By spending our time and energy on intentions rather than actions, we prevent ourselves from living in the now. We lose sight of the only reality we actually have to work with—the present moment.

No regrets from yesterday or desires and anxieties about tomorrow need keep us from our best today.

THOUGHT FOR TODAY: Let us live, let us enjoy, let us create—today.

August 10

The only tyrant I accept in this world is the still small voice within me.

—Mahatma Gandhi

Today my goal will be to keep freedom in the forefront of my consciousness. I will not allow myself to be bound by any limiting thought, attitude, or situation. For the truth is that God has given me absolute and total freedom.

With faith and trust in God's guidance, I can be what I want to be and do what I want to do. No person or circumstance can hinder me from achieving God's will for me. Because of His grace I need not be inhibited or held back by the opinions and perceptions of others. Nor need I be restrained by old ideas and misdirected goals of the past. I have the freedom to set new objectives and do what is necessary to attain them.

Today I will remind myself that God has given me freedom of choice. I will choose to enjoy myself and the company of my friends. I will choose to be positive in my outlook, and to be at ease in all circumstances and situations I may face.

Today I will affirm and accept the many dimensions of my freedom. I will allow freedom to manifest itself within me physically, mentally, emotionally, and spiritually.

THOUGHT FOR TODAY: Personal freedom is an attainable goal.

Who errs and mends, to God himself commends.

—Cervantes

As our understanding of spirituality deepens, we continue to discover new principles and tools. By applying them on a daily basis we are able to enhance our sense of well-being and further our spiritual growth.

One of the most valuable and practical of these tools is a willingness to continually survey our assets and liabilities. We do this for several reasons: to measure progress, to admit and correct our errors, and to avoid a harmful buildup of negative emotions such as anxiety, anger, and fear.

Today when we find that we have been dishonest, irresponsible, or hurtful to others, we quickly try to repair the damage and get back on track. We attempt first to uncover the motives and character flaws behind our behavior. We ask ourselves, for example, if we were being greedy, jealous, or unfair. We then admit our wrongs—to ourselves as well as to those we have harmed—and we set out to correct our errors.

If we do this on a daily basis, we're quickly able to put our problems behind us. As a result we are immeasurably more comfortable. Our relationships are free of tension and hard feelings. We have no secrets—we feel right with ourselves and the world and are able to get on with life.

THOUGHT FOR TODAY: Address today's problems today.

August 12

If we could read the secret history of our enemies, we should find in each man's life sorrow and suffering enough to disarm all hostility.

—Henry Wadsworth Longfellow

Judgmentalism—it can be one of the most unyielding of our character defects. But that's not to say we haven't made a lot of progress. For one thing, we've discovered that we tend to judge in others the very same things we dislike in ourselves. What is more, our growing self-honesty has shown us that being judgmental of another person allows us to feel superior.

We've also learned that this flaw interferes with the development of such qualities as tolerance, understanding, and kindness. That's why it's so important for us to let it go.

In taking steps to do so, it can be extremely helpful to remember that our judgments are usually based on very little information. Most of the time we know hardly anything about the people we are judging. We have no real idea where they come from emotionally, or what they've had to endure and overcome to get where they are now.

So it's really unfair to automatically judge others by our standards; our frame of reference may be totally irrelevant. In fact, it's extremely possible, relatively speaking, that they've made a lot more progress than we have.

THOUGHT FOR TODAY: Our unfair judgments of others are almost always based on too little information.

*Some men can never see an ordinary fact in ordinary terms.
All their geese are swans, until you see the birds.*

—J. B. Owen

These days we don't make a "big deal" out of everything the way we used to. As a result our lives are
much more centered and calm.

It's easy to see now that most big deals were of our
own making and had little or nothing to do with
reality. When we made things larger than life, it was
usually because of our need to feel important—our need
for attention. Besides that, some of us were so hooked
on crisis in our lives that we automatically blew things
out of proportion in order to get our regular "fix" of
adrenaline.

As our attitudes and behavior changed in the areas of
highest priority, it became less important to make a
big deal out of everything. In fact, we had to work
hard at getting rid of our exaggerated perceptions because they interfered greatly with our serenity and
happiness.

Today, there are no big deals because we're learning
to accept things as they are. Moreover, those of us
recovering from addictions simply can't afford big deals
in our lives. We know what's important; we know
where to focus our energies.

THOUGHT FOR TODAY: Today there are no big
deals.

August 14

Perfectionism does not exist; to understand it is the triumph of human intelligence; to expect to possess it is the most dangerous kind of madness.

—Alfred de Musset

My blind pursuit of perfection caused me constant frustration and pain. By trying to achieve the impossible in every area of my life, I set myself up to fail again and again. By demanding perfection in trivial endeavors as well as in matters of consequence, I burned myself out.

Now that I've come to understand my perfectionism and its underlying cause, I've been able to do something about it. What a relief it is to no longer be tyrannized by this self-defeating character flaw.

I still expect a lot from myself. The difference, however, is that I've learned to establish priorities and to seek progress instead of perfection.

Today I evaluate my activities and decide what's really important. I focus my efforts and energies in areas where I know they will make a difference. Specifically, I try to remain self-aware and honest in order to continue building self-esteem. I also put time into cultivating relationships with others, and I try to be more giving. Most important, I work toward spiritual progress by applying the principles I have learned and by seeking conscious contact with God.

THOUGHT FOR TODAY: Focus your energies where you know they will make a difference.

Happiness is not a state to arrive at but a manner of traveling.

—Margaret Lee Runbeck

We tend to look toward certain events for happiness. We're happy when our new car arrives, or when we meet someone special. Vacations bring us happiness, as does recognition in the form of a pay raise or promotion.

That's the way most of us are. The problem is that new cars, vacations, and promotions come into our lives only sporadically. So when we derive happiness mainly from such occurrences, it tends to be an on-again off-again feeling.

But of course happiness need not be limited to specific events or "destinations." There are any number of things we can do to make it a more continuous part of our lives. If we start out with the right attitude, for example, a job well done can bring happiness. Setting new goals or simply being good to ourselves can also be pleasurable. And aren't we happy when we take time to be grateful? Don't we feel good when we do something for someone else?

When we rely on our inner feelings and our actions for happiness, we find that it is with us on a more regular and consistent basis. Happiness is more available to us when we take personal responsibility for it, rather than seek it in outside events.

THOUGHT FOR TODAY: Be responsible for your own happiness.

August 16

The intoxication of anger, like that of the grape, shows us to others, but hides us from ourselves.

—Charles Caleb Colton

Early in my recovery, I was impressed with something I heard about emotional well-being. "Just as your sobriety has followed your drunkenness," a man said, "so will serenity follow your emotional turmoil."

I was comforted by the idea at the time, although I found it hard to imagine that I personally could ever lose my anger. Gradually over the years, however, serenity has indeed begun to replace the rage and resentment that troubled me for so long. I also see parallels between my occasional anger these days and my constant drunkenness of the past. Each is a powerful intoxicant with a high price tag.

When I drank, I usually did so to block out painful feelings. When I become angry, it's often my way to avoid dealing with fear, hurt, or confusion.

When I drank, there was always the strong possibility that I would be locked up in some way. When I become angry, I experience confinement of another sort—the bondage of self.

Whenever I stopped drinking, I went through bone-rattling withdrawal. Similarly, each time I let my anger get out of hand, I experience painful withdrawal in the form of guilt and remorse.

THOUGHT FOR TODAY: When I am angry, I am intoxicated with self.

Lord, deliver me from myself.

—Sir Thomas Browne

On occasion it may seem that our spiritual progress is faltering rather than accelerating as we think it should. We may also feel that our family and friends don't understand or appreciate the new direction our life has been taking. Because we've set our standards and expectations too high, it's possible to end up feeling disappointed by ourselves, other people, and, at certain moments, even by God. We may question the point of following a spiritual path and temporarily lose faith.

When we begin to feel this way, there are several things worth considering. First, we're hardly unique when we experience such doubts. Indeed, religious leaders, prophets, and saints throughout history—Martin Luther, Elijah, and Saint Francis of Assisi, to name a few—acknowledged their own periodic loss of faith and sense of futility.

Even more useful is to remember what our lives used to be like before we acquired faith. Chances are the memories themselves will provide the impetus we need, returning us to a state of gratitude. Finally, we should try to turn our hearts back to God through prayer and meditation. For His power, more than anything, can bring us back from detours of disillusionment to the path of the Spirit.

THOUGHT FOR TODAY: God is always with us, especially when our faith has temporarily faltered.

It is my retreat and resting place from the wars. I try to keep this corner as a haven against the tempest outside, as I do another corner in my soul.

—Michel Eyquem de Montaigne (of his home)

We have repatterned our lives to rid ourselves of self-ishness and other forms of self-centeredness. For we have learned that these traits are at the root of our problems. But we also need to remember that there are things we owe to ourselves. In fact, there are self-oriented actions we must take in order to enhance our self-esteem and bring us closer to God.

We owe ourselves privacy for thought, prayer, and meditation. In order to develop our inner resources and strengthen our relationship with God, we need to set aside peaceful time away from outside pressures.

We need to be good to ourselves in the sense of caring for our physical and emotional health and well-being. This means taking the time and making the effort to exercise, eat right, and get enough rest and recreation—without feeling that we are indulging ourselves.

We also can reserve the right to say no when others urge us to stretch beyond our limits, to participate in actions that could be harmful to us, or to give up the time we have set aside for those things we owe to ourselves and God.

THOUGHT FOR TODAY: Be good to yourself; you deserve it.

Happy is the man who has broken the chains which hurt the mind, and has given up worrying once and for all.

—Ovid

I once attended an art show opening with a friend. When she seemed distracted and unable to concentrate, I asked if anything was the matter. She just had a lot on her mind, she said. Although she hadn't yet started to actually worry, she admitted, she was on the verge.

With a little encouragement my friend described three situations about which she seemed concerned. The auto shop was having difficulty finding a part for her car; she was waiting for the results of a medical test; and there was a rumor at work that the company might be acquired.

"Just getting those things out in the open makes me feel better," my friend said, smiling now. "When we first got to the show it was like there was a rattlesnake in my head. You know, not quite ready to strike, but buzzing away like crazy. And the thing is," she added, "there's absolutely nothing I can do about the car, the test, or the rumor."

We talked for several more minutes and agreed that if there was a common denominator among the three situations, it was certainly her powerlessness over each of them. But there was something she *could* do, we then decided: She could best help herself by letting it all go—and leaving the results up to God.

THOUGHT FOR TODAY: Needless worry can be silenced by accepting the things we cannot change.

August 20

The hopeful man sees success where others see failure, sunshine where others see shadow and storm.

—O. S. Marsden

It's understandable to have regrets about things we've done in the past. We may even wish to shut the door of memory and permanently block out whole periods of our lives. Yet it's possible to become grateful for the past, rather than remain forever penitent. Many of us have been able to turn the seeming liabilities of previous years into useful current assets.

We've learned that this can be done by abandoning our old way of looking at the past, and viewing it with new perspectives that allow us to come to terms with it. We often find that our regretful attitude lies not with the things we actually did, but in the way we feel about those things today.

Perhaps we're still carrying a heavy burden of guilt and have not yet forgiven ourselves. Or maybe we haven't given ourselves enough credit for being disciplined and hardworking as we go about changing old behavior patterns and building new lives.

In my own case, coming to terms with the past took some time. But today I can truly say that I am deeply grateful. By seeking help I not only gained insight into my former problems, but I also was led into an infinitely more rewarding way of living.

THOUGHT FOR TODAY: Yesterday's liabilities can become today's assets.

Ask not that events should happen as you will, but let your will be that events should happen as they do and you shall have peace.

—Epictetus

How will I approach this day? What is my attitude going to be? I have two choices. My actions and reactions can be based on my will—or on God's will.

I know from experience that if I try to do things my way, this day probably will be rough to get through. While I'm trying to control people and situations, I'll be anxious and impatient. And if the results don't meet my expectations, I'll be frustrated and even angry.

If on the other hand I try to align my will with God's will, it's more likely my day will be successful. I'll be better able to accept whatever happens, knowing that everything is as it should be.

Because of my faith and trust in God, I'll be more flexible in my expectations of myself, others, and the day's unfolding events. It's not as likely that I'll be disappointed and upset when things don't go "my way."

Taking this approach, I'll assuredly be more comfortable, calm, and serene throughout the day. With God's guidance, my energy can flow into constructive actions and positive channels instead of being squandered in willful pursuits.

THOUGHT FOR TODAY: Today will be a good day if I try to align my will with God's.

August 22

Learn to say "no"; it will be of more use to you than to be able to read Latin.

—Charles Haddon Spurgeon

Why is it so hard to say no? Why do we so often end up agreeing to do things we don't want to do? Many of us have this problem, and when it happens we become frustrated and even furious with ourselves.

If someone asks us to do something and we say no, we invite their disapproval. We're not anxious to risk anyone's disapproval, especially if we don't have a whole lot of self-esteem to start with. In that sense our inability or unwillingness to say no is out-and-out people-pleasing in one of its most common forms.

If we're tired of allowing our lives to be influenced or controlled by other people's wishes, it's time to take the plunge and learn how to say no. The best way to do it is by starting out in small ways, testing the waters and gradually gaining confidence.

It's helpful to establish priorities and boundaries for ourselves. That way, when we're asked to do something, we'll know in advance how far we're prepared to go. If we're put on the spot, we can give ourselves time to make the decision that's right for us by saying, "Let me think about it."

THOUGHT FOR TODAY: Learning to say no is a function of self-esteem.

That kind of life is most happy which affords us most opportunities of gaining our esteem.

—Samuel Johnson

Looking back from our new vantage point, it's clear to us how we lost what self-esteem we had. Driven by the whiplash of our addictions, many of us compromised our values and morality. Each time we did this by lying, cheating, and misrepresentation, our self-esteem diminished in some way. As our disease progressed, we not only lost sight of the things that once mattered, we also lost ourselves.

In early recovery we were told that the choices we make directly affect the way we feel about ourselves. Since we now have freedom of choice, it was suggested, why not choose to behave and think in ways that make us feel *good* about ourselves?

We tried to do this first by concentrating on restoring our physical health and regaining interest in life. Being honest and respectful to others was also vital to our self-esteem, we soon discovered. With this in mind we set out to rebuild damaged relationships with family, friends, and employers.

By making these and similar choices without compromise, we regain our self-esteem the same way we lost it—one day at a time.

THOUGHT FOR TODAY: The way we feel about ourselves depends greatly on the choices we make.

Si quieres que otro se ría cuenta tus penas, Maria. If you want to make someone laugh, tell him your troubles, Maria.
—Spanish proverb

It's a lot easier to admit we're filled with anger or fear than it is to own up to feeling sorry for ourselves. Self-pity isn't something we're proud of. That's why we tend to hide it, or disguise it as a more respectable emotion. We also deny our self-pity because we know, down deep, that our problems are relatively minor compared to those of other people.

Yet even with this knowledge, we sometimes still exaggerate our woes. Self-pity is seductive; yielding to it seems to take a lot less effort than faith, trust, or positive action. Self-pity is also like quicksand; the longer we wallow in it, the deeper we sink. "Poor me" soon becomes "Why me?" Before long, we're convinced we've been singled out for an inordinate share of adversity.

The simplest way to extricate ourselves from the swamp of self-pity is to firmly acknowledge that we're in it. Talking to a close friend can reinforce our admission, and even help us to laugh about our self-absorption. Of course, the most effective antidote to self-pity is gratitude for the good things in our life, which almost always outweigh the seemingly bad.

THOUGHT FOR TODAY: No matter how bad things seem, self-pity will only make them worse.

Everything that happens in the world is part of a great plan of God running through all time.

—Henry Ward Beecher

It's difficult enough, day by day, to try to envision and understand God's overall plan for us. It's especially hard when tragedies occur, or when we must face major disappointments. How can we learn to accept and deal with unfolding events that are not always to our liking? How can we gain increasing trust in God's sometimes seemingly mysterious ways?

What helps me is to try to change my perspective of myself, acknowledging first that I am but one of millions upon millions of God's children. I stand back and try to see myself and the things that happen in my life as an infinitesimal part of God's limitless and ever-changing universe.

When I get into that meditational frame of mind, I then visualize myself as a small tile—a single tile in a splendid and beautiful mosaic of God's creation.

If I come in really close, focusing only on myself, all I can see is the single tile. However, if I step back and broaden my field of vision, I am able to imagine the entire mosaic in all its glory and perfection. When I can do this, it invariably helps me again to accept myself and what occurs in my life as a necessary part of God's larger plan.

THOUGHT FOR TODAY: You are only one part, but an integral part, of God's glorious mosaic.

August 26

To cheat oneself out of love is the most terrible deception; it is an eternal loss for which there is no reparation, either in time or in eternity.

—Sören Kierkegaard

Life without love seems unimaginable today, but for years that was the reality for many of us. Looking back, we can see that the lack of love in our lives wasn't always due to the inaction of others. Rather, we often deprived ourselves of it.

Although we were unaware at the time, we were actually afraid to have loving relationships. We wouldn't let people get too close because we feared getting hurt in some way. Nor were we able to trust others; we were afraid they might want something from us, or that eventually they would betray our friendship. But more than anything, most of us were unable to accept love because we felt undeserving.

We denied ourselves love for so long that we really didn't know how to let it into our lives. Our relationships with others began to change, however, when we became willing to take small risks. We learned to accept compliments graciously, and tried not to draw back automatically when someone reached out to help us. By allowing ourselves to relate to others, we gradually built rapport. Eventually these bonds of understanding developed into loving relationships.

THOUGHT FOR TODAY: Perhaps the love is there, but we're afraid to let it in.

We cannot conquer fate and necessity, yet we can yield to them in such a manner as to be greater than if we could.
—Walter Savage Landor

The principle of "letting go and letting God" is a keystone of our spiritual beliefs. Yet even after years, many of us still find it difficult to put this concept into practice.

Ironically, the more troubling and persistent a problem is, the harder it is for us to let it go. We're often so emotionally entangled in the situation that we hang on to an old idea: if we try hard enough, *we* can turn it around.

Not only that, we also feel it's our *responsibility* to bring about a solution. We'll admit we're desperate, but what we can't admit—or fail to see—is that in and of ourselves we're powerless to create change.

What usually happens, after pain and frustration have driven us to the wall, is that we finally surrender our will to God's will. We let go and let God. We may still be apprehensive at that point, because we don't know what's going to happen. However, by taking a leap of faith, we've not only opened the door, but also stepped out of the way. We've made it possible for God to provide the solution.

THOUGHT FOR TODAY: Once we stop trying to manage the unmanageable, it becomes possible to "let God."

August 28

Procrastination is the thief of time.

—Edward Young

There's more to procrastination than simply putting things off. If we are to make any real progress in getting rid of this character defect, we first have to become aware of the hidden reasons behind our tendency to procrastinate.

Not surprisingly, fear in various forms is our primary reason for putting things off. We may be fearful of change, or of the unknown. We may be afraid to fail, or to suffer embarrassment. We may have fear of financial insecurity.

We also procrastinate because we'd simply rather do something else—or we're too lazy to do what needs to be done.

Often when we procrastinate, we resort to rationalization to get ourselves off the hook. We try to convince ourselves that we don't have enough time, that we have too many responsibilities, that tomorrow will be soon enough, and so on.

This leads to our procrastination building upon itself, which leads to more procrastination. Before we know it, we can become overwhelmed.

How can we deal constructively with this character defect? Assuming that we already have enough self-awareness and willingness to become rid of our procrastination, we first must uncover and work on the hidden reasons. By taking responsible actions to eliminate the causes of our procrastination, we can eventually become free of the defect itself.

THOUGHT FOR TODAY: To put an end to procrastination, focus first on the hidden causes.

Not knowing when the dawn will come I open every door.
　　　　　　　　　　　　　　—Emily Dickinson

A friend and I were reminiscing about our first year sober. We remembered how tough it was to face problems and experience emotions without being anesthetized in some way. "Those first months were intense," my friend recalled. "I was sure I would drink again. The pain was eating me alive."

For the first time in her life she had to actually face those very same feelings that had caused her to go on benders again and again. "I thought I was going to lose my mind," she said. "All I wanted was to stop feeling bad, but I didn't know what to do. I did know, though, that I couldn't just stay in my room with the door closed."

My friend literally forced herself to talk to other recovering people and tell them how she felt. She was amazed at how much that helped. She sought solutions in books, and tried to vent her feelings in writing. She also tried to stay busy, and found that physical exercise gave her a sense of well-being.

"All those things helped a lot," my friend concluded, "and I still do them today. But more than anything, I believe that God heard me when I asked Him to take away the pain and show me what to do."

THOUGHT FOR TODAY: Open wide your heart and mind, so as to better receive God's grace.

August 30

Much knowledge of things divine escapes us through want of faith.

—Heraclitus

We all know people who live quite adequately without feeling the need to tap spiritual resources. They don't necessarily *disbelieve* in God, nor do they think that faith and trust in a Higher Power is pointless. They simply are satisfied with things as they are and wouldn't have it any other way.

Those of us who now rely on God have no inclination to argue with or proselytize our self-sufficient friends. The great majority of us, in fact, would gladly defend their right to think as they wish. We've gotten out of the habit of judging others.

But since discovering the rewards of faith, we too wouldn't have it any other way. For we experience every aspect of our lives in entirely different and more satisfying ways than when we relied solely on our own resources.

Unrestricted by limiting thoughts and attitudes, we now enjoy freer and more expansive lives. Each day we are renewed with enthusiasm and joy. Because we know that God is with us now and forever, our fears have diminished greatly. As we turn to His care, He calms and sustains us.

Never again need we feel alone or friendless. Regardless of the confusion and discord around us, God keeps us serene and peaceful. He is our constant source of strength, assurance, and comfort.

THOUGHT FOR TODAY: Remember the rewards of faith.

Maturity of mind is the capacity to endure uncertainty.
                                        —John Finley

You look at your watch and figure the time difference between the East and West coasts. Another business day has passed, and you still don't know whether your grant has been approved. You curse and shake your head angrily as you storm out of the house.

We've all been there—we know what it's like to go through periods of uncertainty. Yet some of us have to be reminded over and over that the way we feel during these ordeals is largely up to us. The important thing is how we react; the person or institution that is keeping us dangling is almost irrelevant.

If this is a period of uncertainty for us, now is the perfect time to step back and examine the only two choices we have. One, of course, is to fume and fret. But if we choose to do that we know from experience that we'll likely become more angry, fearful, or even obsessed.

The far more mature choice is to look at and accept the reality of the situation, realizing that any number of possibilities could explain a delay in learning the outcome of something. In the meantime, we have to go on with our lives, trying to keep faith in this idea: Things will turn out the way they're supposed to, but only *when* they're supposed to.

THOUGHT FOR TODAY: Choose to be emotionally sober during times of uncertainty.

September 1

If you wish to drown, do not torture yourself with shallow water.

—Bulgarian proverb

I sometimes think of my life as existing in three "realms" —dry land, shallow water, and the deep. When I'm on dry land, I'm thinking straight, doing what's good and right, and taking the actions that have proved to be valuable in building a life of faith and happiness.

When I plunge into the deep—for whatever reason —I'm quickly swept away and overcome by negative thinking, old ideas, and destructive behavior. There's no question from the first instant that I'm in great jeopardy.

The danger is almost as great, however, when I move into shallow water, that seductive and deceptively secure middle area. For me as an addictive person, "moving into shallow water" means flirting with dangerous thoughts and behavior. When I move into shallow water I toy with insanity by asking myself, "Should I, or shouldn't I . . . ?" Shallow water is torturous, most certainly, but more importantly for me it's also a sure pathway to disaster.

On that day when I find myself heading away from dry land and toward the deep—on that day when the shallow water seems especially inviting—I will ask God to restore me to sanity and will trust in His power to do so.

THOUGHT FOR TODAY: If you don't want to slip, don't give power to slippery thoughts.

To will what God wills is the only science that gives us rest.
—Henry Wadsworth Longfellow

God has given us vital personal resources with which to live our lives. He also has given us the free will to use them as we choose. We have been given intelligence, judgment, and the power to reason.

Looking back, we can see that most of our problems resulted from our misuse of these resources. Our intelligence was inhibited by our tendency to delude ourselves. Our judgment was distorted by resentment and low self-esteem. Our power to reason was weakened by the intensity of our emotional involvements. But it was our overriding self-centeredness, more than anything, that caused our difficulties.

When we turned our lives over to the care of God, it became a lot easier to make right choices and live successfully. As we grew less self-centered and more open-minded, our entire perspective on life changed. We were better able to think honestly, to judge fairly, and to reason clearly. By relying on God for guidance and strength, we gradually learned how to effectively apply our tools for living.

THOUGHT FOR TODAY: God provides the blueprint, the tools, and the power; the rest is up to us.

September 3

Friendship either finds or makes equals.

—Publilius Syrus

We didn't fit in—that was one of our most pervasive feelings. No matter where we were, or whom we were with, we felt awkward and different. Moreover, we were convinced we were the only ones in the world who had such feelings. We believed we would go through our entire lives with a sense of aloneness.

When we became willing to break out of our isolation, we found we had been quite mistaken. By risking more open communication, we discovered with enormous relief that others had felt exactly as we did.

At first we had to force ourselves to share at levels deeper than those surface ones that always had been safest and most comfortable. But as soon as we took that risk, we experienced dramatic changes in the way we felt when we were around other people. By relating our long-hidden feelings, and identifying with those shared by others, we began to have a real sense of belonging.

For the first time in our lives, we focused on the similarities rather than the differences between ourselves and others. We know now that although we are unique as individuals, in the final analysis we are not really that different from other people.

THOUGHT FOR TODAY: Look for the similarities, not the differences.

Miracles are instantaneous—they cannot be summoned, but come of themselves, usually at unlikely moments and to those who least expect them.

—Katherine Anne Porter

A year or so into my sobriety, I was still struggling to fully overcome my atheism. During that period I went through an extremely traumatic personal experience. It brought me frighteningly close to drinking. For two days I forgot all about the principle of "surrendering to win." I clenched my fists, relying on willpower to overcome an irresistible desire to get drunk. I knew that if I did drink I would likely die, but I was at the point where I didn't care.

In desperation I called a friend. "I know you don't believe in God," he said, "but that's the only thing that works for me. I'd pray for God to take away the compulsion."

I got down on my knees and asked for God's help— even though I didn't have much faith in what I was doing. Later that evening, still close to the edge, I pulled my car into a covered parking place. Slouched in a corner not far from me, a man was drinking from a pint bottle of wine. He was drunk and sick, and he looked enough like me to be my twin brother. When I finally stopped staring and turned away, my desire to drink had been lifted.

That miracle saved my life. I realize, looking back, that it also was the starting point for my faith.

THOUGHT FOR TODAY: Coincidences are sometimes miracles of God, who prefers to remain anonymous.

September 5

Anyone can carry his burden, however heavy, until nightfall.
Anyone can do his work, however hard, for one day.
— Robert Louis Stevenson

There are times when we face especially difficult tasks. When we contemplate the enormity of what lies ahead, our projections often tell us that we can't possibly make it through—even though we must. We can become so thoroughly persuaded we're going to fall short, that our negative conviction becomes a self-fulfilling prophecy.

Before we get to that point, it may be helpful to mentally step outside of the situation—to change perspective as well as develop a better game plan. It may also be useful simply to think about how we actually live our lives. If we take a moment to do that, it becomes quickly obvious that few things are accomplished all at once. We eat our meals one bite at a time, we drive to work one mile at a time, our lifeblood is pumped one heartbeat at a time.

If all of this is true, why then do we sometimes feel we have to take on life's difficult challenges in their entirety? The point is that we don't have to. We can accomplish even the most burdensome tasks one day at a time—or, if that's too much, one hour or even one minute at a time.

THOUGHT FOR TODAY: Negative projections can become self-fulfilling prophecies.

Fire and sword are but slow engines of destruction in comparison with the babbler.

—Sir Richard Steele

Our emotional sobriety depends in large measure on avoiding behavior that could be hurtful to others. We know from experience what turmoil we create within ourselves when we lose our tempers, are overly critical of others, or simply act unfairly.

But what about forms of behavior that are less obvious? Gossip is a primary case in point. When we gossip about someone behind his or her back, our "disclosures" invariably are personal, intimate, and of a sensational nature. And although the information we pass along may be based on fact, most often it is exaggerated or groundless. In any case, gossip by its nature is always malicious and hurtful, no matter what our intentions or rationalizations.

We gossip because we get something out of it. By spreading a belittling rumor about another person, aren't we trying to make ourselves look better in comparison? For some, gossip is a sick form of entertainment. For all, it is a sign of insecurity.

Before we say something malicious about another person, we might think ahead of time of the consequences that will follow. We will surely hurt the person about whom we're gossiping—and we will hurt those we're dragging into our "confidence." But most of all, we will hurt ourselves.

THOUGHT FOR TODAY: No matter what the motive, gossip is always hurtful to all concerned.

September 7

It is good for us to think no grace or blessing truly ours, till we are aware that God has blessed someone else with it through us.

—Phillips Brooks

From the very first days that we welcomed God into our lives, His grace was evident to us through the actions of others. When we were most alone, we were offered friendship. When we needed help, it was soon at hand. When we were lost, we were shown the way.

In a short time we were ready to pass along God's grace. By reaching out to those in need, we became a channel for His spirit, which we believe flows through us and into the lives of others.

There were times, even during the darkest days of the past, when we secretly wished we could somehow be givers rather than takers. But it was not until our spirit became harmonious with God's spirit that we were able to give freely, and to reap the indescribable rewards of doing so.

Today we pray that we can be free of self, in order to become a clear channel for God's spirit. We pray that His love will flow through us into the lives of others.

THOUGHT FOR TODAY: By reaching out to others in harmony with God, I can become a channel for His grace.

This is certain, that a man that studieth revenge keeps his wounds green, which otherwise would heal and do well.
—Francis Bacon

I've learned that when I'm seriously upset I have to quickly quiet the disturbance, no matter who or where I think it comes from. This is especially true when I resent someone or something.

When I'm seething with resentment, I'm the one who suffers. That suffering can take various self-destructive forms. I almost always become obsessed, losing whatever serenity and comfort I may have. All I can think of are the ways in which I've been hurt—and the ways by which I can retaliate. Consequently, my "right now" becomes ruined and I begin to edge God out of my life.

Resentments also distort my thinking, causing me to do things harmful to those around me and myself.

Perhaps most dangerous, my priorities go awry. I revert to my old ways of handling situations. And when this happens I'm in great danger of forgetting the things that must come first in my life.

When I find myself getting upset, will I pause and try to remember what happens to me when I allow myself to get carried away?

THOUGHT FOR TODAY: Quiet the disturbance; remember the priorities.

September 9

The breeze of divine grace is blowing upon us all. But one needs to set the sail to feel the breeze of grace.

—Ramakrishna

When we take our first faltering steps on the road to recovery, we hope for little else than to be relieved of our self-destructive thoughts and behavior. With God's help, this soon occurs for many of us.

For a time we are content, but then one day an intriguing possibility is presented. If by God's power we've been granted a release from our obsessions and addictions, why shouldn't we by the same means be able to achieve a release from other difficulties, such as jealousy, depression, and fear?

Certainly we had tried long enough and hard enough to change ourselves through our own efforts—with little or no success. So what did we have to lose?

Little by little, we tried to employ God's power and grace in other areas of our lives. Gradually, things changed for the better. Our faith deepened and our trust grew stronger. And eventually we found ourselves presenting to others the same intriguing possibility that had been presented to us.

How exactly can we "set our sail" to make the possibility a reality? We must be truly aware that a particular character flaw isn't working; we must become ready and willing to have it removed; we must humbly ask God to remove it.

THOUGHT FOR TODAY: Expect a miracle, but do the footwork.

Some of the best lessons we ever learn, we learn from our mistakes and failures. . . . The error of the past is the wisdom and success of the future.

—Tryon Edwards

It's impossible to live in the world and not make mistakes; everyone knows that. What we sometimes forget is that we need to decide what to do *after* we make the mistake. We can act in ways that compound the original error, or we can take constructive action. The choice is ours.

We all know people who quickly acknowledge their mistakes with profuse apologies. But nothing really changes; they go on repeating the same mistakes over and over again.

Then there are those who react pridefully. They defend their actions, make excuses, and constantly seek ways to justify themselves. The upshot is that they stubbornly refuse to admit their mistakes and change their ways.

Some people, when they make mistakes, can't or won't forgive themselves. They seek punishment and become their own lifelong victims.

We've all made at least one of these poor choices in dealing with mistakes. Each time we've done so, it's become clear that there are better ways. By personally acknowledging and accepting the mistake, we can more easily admit it to someone else. We can then apologize or make amends. By learning as much as we can from the error, chances are we won't be doomed to repeat it.

THOUGHT FOR TODAY: What we do *after* we make a mistake is more important than the original error.

September 11

Nothing in life is more remarkable than the unnecessary anxiety which we endure, and generally occasion ourselves.
—Benjamin Disraeli

I'm grateful for the many ways in which my perceptions and reactions have taken 180-degree turns. Time, for example—something as basic as that—used to be a major source of anxiety in my life.

I owned several watches and insisted on keeping a clock in every room, but that was the least of it. Because of my irresponsible actions, I was always late for appointments. I missed not only airplanes but also deadlines; toward the end I was too sick to even try to be on time.

Because of my thinking, I would put imaginary time restraints on myself. One constant refrain, I remember, went something like this: "By this time I should have been . . . By this time I should have had . . . By this time I should have done . . ."

If I had three hours in which to complete an assignment, instead of saying, "I have three hours, that's great!" I would say, "I only have three hours, that's terrible!"

Looking back, perhaps it was all a way of keeping things stirred up. By creating a constant atmosphere of crisis, I was able for a long time to avoid confronting my real problems.

THOUGHT FOR TODAY: Hard time or easy time, good time or bad time—it's up to you.

Peace is when time doesn't matter when it passes by.
—Maria Schell

Time was my enemy, but now it has become my friend. In the old days, I used to constantly berate myself because I hadn't achieved a certain goal or amassed a certain sum of money by a certain time. When I became sick and tired of making impossible demands on myself, I was able to eliminate much of that time-related anxiety. Eventually I learned that all I have to do is the best I'm able to do, and trust God to do the rest.

I no longer feel imprisoned by time, and now see it for what it is—simply a numerical system designed to help me rather than torment me. Consequently I've learned to use time to my advantage—I'm free to organize it, schedule it, or even to disregard it.

Because I'm not stress-ridden these days, I'm able to use my time more efficiently. It's easier to concentrate on what I'm doing—I make fewer mistakes, I'm more relaxed, and my friends say it's often a pleasure being around me.

I find that pretty amazing. The thing is, time is the same now as it's always been—sixty minutes in an hour, twenty-four hours in a day. Time hasn't changed, but clearly *I* have.

THOUGHT FOR TODAY: Everything in God's time.

September 13

Care is no cure, but rather corrosive for things that are not to be remedied.

—William Shakespeare

At some time in our lives we are bound to get involved with friends or family members whose behavior is harmful to themselves or others. Perhaps a brother, sister, spouse, or parent is a practicing alcoholic whose illness is killing him or her and wreaking havoc in the lives of everyone around him or her. Perhaps a friend continually puts himself or herself in danger because of sexual promiscuity. Or maybe a person with whom we're close is putting his career at risk and himself in personal jeopardy as a result of his questionable business practices.

Because we care, we do everything we can to make these persons aware of what they're doing. We express concern, and offer assistance if that's indicated. But if they choose to or are compelled to continue along their destructive paths, there's nothing more we can do other than release them with love and pray for their well-being.

As we all know, this is extremely difficult to do; it never seems to get any easier. Yet if we honestly recognize and accept our powerlessness—and put our faith in God's power—we find that's the best possible thing we can do for all concerned.

THOUGHT FOR TODAY: When you release someone with love, you free yourself.

Prayer is not eloquence, but earnestness; not definition of hopelessness, but the feeling of it; not figures of speech, but earnestness of soul.

—Hannah More

Sometimes we forget the purpose of prayer. We may feel inhibited and even self-conscious in reaction to the eloquence of familiar spiritual personalities. Or perhaps we feel that our prayers don't measure up to classic prayers in religious services or inspirational literature. For these and other reasons, we may feel on occasion that we're "not doing a good job" in communicating with our Higher Power.

When we begin to think like this, we can remind ourselves why we pray and what it has done for us. In my own case, I began praying in desperation, out of a sense of utter helplessness. My initial prayers were little more than pleas to God for an end to pain.

Although my prayers never have become "articulate," they have become calmer and more sincere. They are offered not only during periods of crisis, but on a regular basis each day, more often as an expression of gratitude than of suffering.

What I have learned over time is that the purpose of my prayers is to concede my powerlessness, while reaffirming my faith and trust in God's power. My prayers are not always answered right away, but I invariably feel relief—in the form of altered consciousness—almost instantly.

THOUGHT FOR TODAY: Pray this day for knowledge of God's will, and for ever stronger trust in Him.

September 15

Fear is the darkroom in which all of your negatives are developed.

—Unknown

When we are fearful, it often seems that our feelings have come out of nowhere. The reality, however, is that fear is not an abstract emotion. Fears arise from such things as memories of painful experiences, feelings of inadequacy, or simply our tendency to project the worst rather than the best. Our egos are a primary breeding ground for our fears. In fact, ego and fear are more closely related than is readily apparent.

Some people, for example, have long been interested in learning a new sport. Yet they've never done anything about it because of their fear. It's not that they're afraid of the sport per se, but rather that they'll injure themselves while learning, or that others will laugh at their amateurish efforts.

In such situations, we can't simply decide not to be fearful. What we can do, though, is to approach our irrational fears in rational ways. One way is to walk into fear's "darkroom" and take a good look at all those negatives. When we do that, we'll find that we're not seeing reality at all, but pure ego projection. We'll realize that when we let fear hold us back, we're allowing our egos, rather than our hearts and minds, to make choices for us.

THOUGHT FOR TODAY: Fears are negatives that need not be developed.

There are people who always find a hair in their plate of soup for the simple reason that, when they sit down before it, they shake their head until one falls in.

—Friedrick Hebbel

One measure of positive growth in my life is that it's not so easy anymore to blame my troubles on other people. It's become quite difficult, in fact, to insist and truly believe that I'm a "victim of circumstances."

There was a time when just the opposite was true. If I was pulled over for drunk driving, I'd automatically reason that the police were out to get me because I was driving a sports car. If that dentist hadn't given me pain pills, I wouldn't have become addicted. If they hadn't served champagne at my brother's wedding, I wouldn't have ended up in jail.

Now that I'm living in reality, such attitudes seem far-fetched—sometimes even amusing. I have to remember, though, that they were hardly funny at the time—I was seriously deluded. I also need to remember that it's possible for me to slip back into those attitudes, and that as a result my life would go downhill faster than I can imagine.

Do I see now that only I am responsible for what happens to me when I make a choice or take an action? Am I willing to continue to take responsibility?

THOUGHT FOR TODAY: I am responsible for my own actions and the consequences thereof.

September 17

Any fool can carry on, but only the wise man knows how to shorten sail.

—Joseph Conrad

Our serenity comes in large measure from our willingness to adapt to the ever-changing cadence of life. That's why we're striving to be increasingly flexible in our approach to all things.

If, for example, we are willing to change speed, procedure, or even direction at work when major changes are underway, we will be better able to face emerging challenges or to take advantage of new opportunities. When we are involved in a project with other people, our flexibility and open-mindedness will allow us to be more cooperative and considerate. Our interactions will become more pleasant, and everyone will benefit.

When we are willing to take time out to evaluate and adapt to changing circumstances at home—the birth of a child, for example, or the necessity for major financial adjustments—we will be better prepared to contribute to the health and stability of our family relationships.

If, on the other hand, we dig in our heels and insist on continuing to do things our way, we are far more likely to feel pressured, to lose our serenity, and ultimately, to be defeated by our own inflexibility.

THOUGHT FOR TODAY: The more mentally flexible we can be, the more tranquility we are likely to have.

Never be afraid of giving up your best, and God will give you His better.

—James Hinton

The spiritual principle of surrender has become a keystone of our lives. We have discovered that when we surrender, God will do for us what we cannot do for ourselves. But what are the dynamics of this principle? What actually happens?

The first thing that must occur is for us to reach bottom—to become sick and tired of whatever it is that has been making us sick and tired: a character defect, an old idea, an unhealthy relationship, an obsession, or an illness—relatively minor problems as well as serious ones.

Following that, we must accept our powerlessness, conceding that it is futile to keep fighting the person, place, or thing causing us difficulty. We must also concede that it is beyond our capability to "fix" the situation. We admit that we need help from a Power greater than ourselves.

What usually happens at this point is that the negative feelings that have festered within us—anger, resentment, fear and, above all, frustration—become greatly diminished. Because we have stopped trying to do things our way and have begun to approach the situation calmly, it becomes possible for God to enter our life and bring about change.

THOUGHT FOR TODAY: When we surrender spiritually, God does for us what we cannot do for ourselves.

September 19

My body is that part of the world which my thoughts can alter. Even imaginary illnesses can become real ones. In the rest of the world my hypotheses cannot disturb the order of things.

—George Christoph Lichtenberg

Because of the way I used to live, illnesses and accidents were commonplace. Because of the way I thought and felt, I invariably played up the seriousness of my condition. At the time, my denial of many things was so strong that I wasn't aware I was doing anything out of the ordinary. But I can see now that such behavior was an illness unto itself—I had a sick need to be sick.

Why did I exaggerate my ailments? So people wouldn't expect so much from me. So I could get more of the attention I constantly craved. So I could feel sorry for myself and thereby justify continuing to think and act in the same self-destructive ways.

When I think back to those days of real and imagined ailments, I'm grateful for numerous things. First, I've drastically changed my life-style, so I don't get sick or hurt as often as I used to. Second, when I do get sick I don't immediately indulge myself with self-pity; I see my illness for what it is and take care of it sensibly. Finally, I've been able to develop new attitudes that can sometimes alter the course of an illness in positive rather than negative ways.

THOUGHT FOR TODAY: Cherish the healing light.

The bitter and the sweet come from the outside, the hard from within, from one's own efforts.

—Albert Einstein

When success or personal triumphs come our way, we may need to exercise special caution. For we have found that good fortune can put us in a precarious frame of mind. We can quickly lose whatever emotional sobriety and humility we have gained over time.

All too often in the past, we had as much trouble dealing with success as with seeming failure. When we experienced good fortune, we often blew it and ourselves way out of proportion. We immediately craved even greater success and, in no time at all, exhibited all the emotional trappings of our illusory sense of power.

We became arrogant, manipulative, and uncaring. Not surprisingly, our behavior turned people off and, ultimately, turned them away. Then we were left feeling empty and alone.

Those are some of the emotional pitfalls we try to avoid today. But what helps us keep proper perspective, more than anything, is this realization: Any success we have today is far more God's doing than our own. Our personal triumphs or achievements do not in any way change the balance of power between ourselves and Him.

THOUGHT FOR TODAY: In most respects we are powerless; in every respect God has all power.

September 21

There is no heavier burden than an unfulfilled potential.
— Charles Schulz

When we begin to enjoy the rewards of right living and right thinking, we experience many freedoms. We have the freedom to choose new friends and a new life-style. We have the freedom to put aside or reject old habits and ideas.

An especially gratifying freedom for some of us is no longer having to buy into the idea that we're "not living up to our potential." This message may have been subtly transmitted by employers and friends, or constantly drummed into us by family members. For the most part, however, we were the ones who burdened ourselves with the notions that we weren't where we should have been—we weren't doing what we were capable of doing—or we hadn't progressed far enough.

The difference today is our self-awareness. Now that we know who we are, what we want, and what our capabilities and limitations are, we've begun to lose many of our insecurities. We've become less vulnerable to outside pressure, and are less likely to react defensively when people or our own self-destructive ideas try to convince us we're not living up to our potential.

THOUGHT FOR TODAY: The more self-aware you become, the freer you are to make your own choices.

Nature is the living, visible garment of God.

—Goethe

Autumn has arrived and the air is sharp with the scent of impending change. We are certain now that summer's heat will finally give way to invigorating days and crisp nights, and we are relieved.

At times it is the same with our lives. Just when we feel that we have had quite enough—*more* than enough—of certain situations or stages, God surprises us by bringing about change and relief miraculously, as only He can do.

Not long ago it seemed that summer would never end. Then we awakened one morning to find the hillsides vibrant with the colors of early autumn. We looked skyward and saw formations of migrating birds, their journeys to warmer climates already begun.

When we think about our life, we see that it too has its "seasons." The changes may not be as regular or predictable as the passage from summer to fall or fall to winter, but they are no less momentous. When we review the changes that have already taken place within us and about us, we are filled with excitement and hope for the changes to come.

THOUGHT FOR TODAY: Now that I am on the right path, I welcome continuing change in my life.

September 23

The most important thought I ever had was that of my individual responsibility to God.

—Daniel Webster

I was told at the start of my recovery that if I was to remain sober and live comfortably, I would have to apply spiritual principles in my life. From my own direct experience I know that these principles work.

When I regularly and consistently practice patience, tolerance, and understanding, I am at peace with myself and the world around me. When I revert to my old ways of impatience, intolerance, and selfishness, I find I can't afford the high price I must pay for such behavior.

Over time the practice of these principles has taken on deeper meaning and greater value. Today I try to live on a spiritual plane not only because there's really no other way for me, but also because that life-style enables me to express gratitude to God for His many gifts: sobriety, freedom, happiness, friendship, and the opportunity to be of service to others.

The best possible way for me to thank God for His blessings is to bring the principles I have learned into all my relationships and activities.

THOUGHT FOR TODAY: Your sobriety is God's gift to you. What you do with your sobriety is your gift to God.

In character, in manners, in style, in all things, the supreme excellence is simplicity.

—Henry Wadsworth Longfellow

We fancied ourselves as complicated people. Certainly our approach to most things was complicated. Even when we faced simple problems, we usually dealt with them in convoluted and complex ways. We'd run ourselves ragged before finally coming around to the simple solutions we had overlooked from the start.

Some of us carried this approach into recovery. When simple solutions were offered, we tended to apply them in complicated ways. It was suggested, for example, that we make a written self-examination. We spun our wheels for months, agonizing over *how, where,* and *when.* In the end we realized that if we had kept it simple—concentrating on the purpose rather than the method—we would have saved ourselves a great deal of frustration and anxiety.

Gradually, we learned the value of simplicity. We saw not only that our complicated approach was a waste of time, but also that it delayed our progress in almost every area of our lives. Today in personal relationships, in the work area, and in our application of spiritual principles, we are most successful when we keep it simple.

THOUGHT FOR TODAY: Simple solutions work best for "complicated" people.

September 25

Oftentimes nothing profits more than self-esteem, grounded on what is just and right.

—John Milton

When we first heard the expression "self-love," we couldn't relate to it very well. We were so used to thinking harshly of ourselves that it was difficult to imagine a gentler point of view. Besides that, we weren't even sure we wanted to love ourselves; there seemed something almost distasteful about the notion.

To make matters worse, we were getting contradictory messages. On the one hand, self-love was presented to us as a worthy and attainable goal. On the other, we were advised that we would have to become rid of self in *all* its forms in order to make spiritual progress.

But once we got past the semantics, it became clear that there are two sides to self-love. There is the destructive side, from which we suffered most of our lives. Born of our egocentricity, it insisted that we were not only unique and superior, but always right.

The other side of self-love—for which we now strive—flows from a true awareness and complete acceptance of who we are. It reflects a willingness to be equal with others, as well as a healthy and realistic sense of human dignity.

THOUGHT FOR TODAY: We gain self-love by becoming free of self.

Friendship improves happiness, and abates misery, by doubling our joy, and dividing our grief.

—Joseph Addison

There is no question that we feel better and "do" better when we regularly interact with others. Life is so much richer when we have friends with whom we can share our joys and troubles. Unfortunately, though, loneliness remains a major problem and source of pain for many. But none of us need become resigned to loneliness, because loneliness is completely "treatable," if not actually avoidable.

The first, most important thing we can do for ourselves is to admit frankly that we're troubled by our loneliness. Writing about our living patterns and feelings certainly can be useful in that regard. The next step is deciding to actually do something about it. At this point it can be helpful to confide in someone we trust, and perhaps receive some suggestions.

Those of us who have overcome loneliness were most successful when we made a real effort to reach out to others. When we "put out our hand" and started conversations, we were quickly encouraged by the responsiveness of most people.

Many of us broke through our isolation by participating in activities that involved being around people. We signed up for classes and met new friends while learning a hobby, sport, or language.

THOUGHT FOR TODAY: Loneliness is not only "treatable," but avoidable.

September 27

Jealousy sees things always with magnifying glasses which make little things large, of dwarfs giants, of suspicions truths.

—Cervantes

Following the death of his parents, a friend of mine inherited a substantial fortune. Several months later, he described some of the ways in which his life had begun to change. He prefaced his story by telling me that he had been a very jealous person. When he became wealthy he had the opportunity to see the emotion clearly for the first time, through the behavior of two lifelong friends.

The first one was sincerely caring and understanding; that was evident by his attitude and actions. "He realized I was going through big emotional changes, and he was supportive and helpful. But nothing in our basic relationship changed. He treated me the same as before, which I really appreciated."

The second person was extremely jealous of my friend's wealth. He became slightly antagonistic, and frequently made sardonic remarks about his own need to "watch every penny." Where before the relationship had been easy and warm, it grew cool and tense.

"The main thing I noticed," my friend said, "was how much *he* was suffering because of his jealousy. I saw myself reflected in him, and I felt badly for him, because I knew exactly how he felt."

THOUGHT FOR TODAY: When you see a character flaw in another, learn what you can from it—about yourself.

We need the faith to go a path untrod, the power to be alone and vote with God.

—Edward Markham

More and more these days I intuitively know how to handle situations that used to baffle me. When I find myself with a person who is suffering, for example, I seem to know what to say and how to act in order to be helpful. Or when I'm confronted with unforeseen events—be they minor mishaps or major calamities—I don't fall apart or flounder as I used to, but instead usually know what to do.

There's no question in my mind why this has come about. It's the direct result of my willingness to live a spiritual life—to seek God's guidance and wisdom each day, to ask Him to direct my thoughts and actions.

By practicing these spiritual principles over a period of time, my sense of what is good, right, and necessary has evolved and become an integral part of me. The more I am able to follow this intuition and to experience its benefits, the greater is my trust in God and the less I tend to rely solely on my own limited resources.

How much easier and more comfortable life has become because of this. How much better I get along with others. How much happier I am!

THOUGHT FOR TODAY: As faith and trust in God grow, so does intuition.

September 29

Whatever the universal nature assigns to any man at any time is for the good of that man at that time.
—Marcus Aurelius

It can take a long time and severe discomfort before we become willing to make major changes in our lives. When we finally do take the first step, we're often so eager for immediate results that we become impatient if things don't happen as quickly as we would like them to.

Is it possible that we grow impatient and frustrated because we're tackling our new goals with the same old and ineffective tools we've always used—self-will, perfectionism, and the expectation of instant success?

What we really should do is approach these goals with keen-edged new tools and attitudes—acceptance and patience to begin with, followed by the willingness to take action one day at a time even when results aren't readily apparent.

Above all, we need to remember that no one can turn around his or her entire life overnight. Not only is that an unattainable goal, it's also an extremely burdensome one. If we're to be successful at changing, we should try to understand that progress usually comes gradually—and we should count on the fact that it will occasionally be interrupted by seeming setbacks.

THOUGHT FOR TODAY: Seek progress, not perfection.

God planted fear in the soul as truly as He planted hope or courage. It is a kind of bell or gong which rings the mind into quick life and avoidance on the approach of danger. It is the soul's signal for rallying.

—Henry Ward Beecher

One of our first clear-headed awarenesses in recovery is the destructive role of fear in our lives. It is surprising and dismaying to see how this tyrannical emotion has influenced practically every thought and action. We soon learn that freedom from fear is a lifetime undertaking, one that can never be entirely completed.

Yet for all its usual damaging effects, fear can lead us on to better things. Fear of disaster and self-destruction, for example, forced us to embrace a solution to our addictions. In recovery, we're mainly motivated to do the right thing—to be honest, kind, and tolerant—because we want to, and in order to grow spiritually. But here again fear can be a motivating force when we're afraid of the consequences of being *dis*honest, *un*kind, and *in*tolerant.

Perhaps paradoxically, fear brings many of us to the doorstep of faith—to the beginning of belief in a Power greater than ourselves. Each time we turn to God when we are fearful or uncertain, our faith is strengthened. And as our faith grows, our fears are lessened.

THOUGHT FOR TODAY: Sometimes fear can be turned to our advantage, motivating us to do what is right and necessary.

October 1

*What is a cynic? A man who knows the price of everything
and the value of nothing.*

—Oscar Wilde

I used to pride myself on my cynicism. By relying on
this way of relating to other people and the world in
general, I was able to feel clever, unique, and sneer-
ingly superior.

Although I realize that cynicism is a valued form of
expression in certain circles and can be the basis for humor,
in my own life the consequences were neither valuable nor
humorous. Cynicism as I practiced it was a harmful character defect born out of low self-esteem and fear.

I know now that my cynicism was a major defense
mechanism—a way to keep people from getting too
close. My "know-it-all" judgments of everything and
everybody served as armor that protected me from
emotional involvement. But they also deprived me of
the values of human experience.

Since I so often tried to pass myself off as an expert,
my mind was usually locked tight. It was almost impossible for me to learn or try anything new. This was
especially true for ideas and objectives of a spiritual
nature. Consequently, cynicism blocked me off from
God for many years.

When I occasionally become cynical today, I have to
remind myself not to take this character flaw lightly.
For me cynicism is not a stylish game, but is always
seriously consequential, with all penalties and no rewards.

THOUGHT FOR TODAY: The behavioral armor that
protects, also deprives.

The sun, with all those planets revolving around it and dependent on it, can still ripen a bunch of grapes as if it had nothing else in the universe to do.

—Galileo Galilei

On our busier days it's easy to get caught up in responsibilities, focusing only on what *we* have to do. We become distanced from others and isolated in our own little worlds. There's just not enough time, we say, to respond to messages on our answering machines, to see how friends are, to be kind to people with whom we come in contact.

Yet no matter how busy we may be, it's still essential to keep our priorities in order. We need to find the time, or make the time, to reach out to others in whatever ways we can.

"Being there" for other people will always remain a top priority in our lives. For one thing, we've learned that we have to "give it away to keep it." For another, we don't want to take our blessings for granted; we want to keep in mind how much it means to us when a kind or encouraging word comes our way.

When we are generous of spirit, it's difficult to remain self-involved. That being the case, the way we interact with others can truly change the complexion of the day. And besides, we feel so much better about ourselves when we've made an effort to be kind and caring.

THOUGHT FOR TODAY: Considering the importance of kindness, are we ever too busy to be kind?

October 3

Life must be understood backwards. But it must be lived forwards.

—Sören Kierkegaard

Only when we came to terms with the past and were willing to learn from it could we move freely forward. Once we became aware of this, we were anxious to embark on a journey of discovery.

First, we took an honest and revealing look at both our past and present. We put our findings on paper to more clearly see patterns of behavior that caused us difficulty. Many of us were able to see for the first time what "people-pleasers" we were, for example, or the extent to which fear ruled our lives.

In order to unburden ourselves of our "secrets," and to make a start at gaining humility, we shared what we had written with someone we trusted. Once that person helped us identify our major character flaws, we were usually quite willing to be free of them. We were told that we couldn't "will" them away, but that God could and would remove them if we asked Him. Next we set out to offer amends for our wrongs. Where we could, we repaired damaged relationships.

If we have been honest and diligent in our "house-cleaning," we've already begun to receive benefits. We've been able to shed a great deal of guilt. We've learned to forgive ourselves. We've also discovered a set of spiritual tools that actually work, and can be applied and reapplied in our daily lives.

THOUGHT FOR TODAY: Reconciling with the past helps us live comfortably in the now.

Ewig ist ein langer Kauf. Forever is a long bargain.
—German proverb

The morning after the first time I got drunk, I swore that I would never drink again. I was only twelve years old. Over the next several decades this routine was to be repeated countless times—I got drunk and swore off, I got drunk and swore off, *ad infinitum*.

During those years my disease progressed relentlessly. From time to time I became very ill or got into serious trouble. On those occasions I vowed to quit forever.

The last time that I swore off, I was offered help by a recovering alcoholic who seemed to know exactly what I was going through. When I expressed doubts that this time would be different, explaining that I had always failed when I had quit in the past, he offered a suggestion that changed my life.

My new friend told me that "forever" is too long a time for an alcoholic to stay away from alcohol; the very idea is as impossible to imagine as it is to undertake. But we can stay sober for one day, he said. That's the way we do it—we don't drink today, and we deal with tomorrow when it arrives.

THOUGHT FOR TODAY: Don't take the first drink or pill—today. Worry about tomorrow—tomorrow.

October 5

The more faithfully you listen to the voice within you, the better you will hear what is sounding outside. And only he who listens can speak.

—Dag Hammarskjöld

On occasion we may feel uncomfortable around other people, especially in social situations. We walk into a room and everyone looks great: they seem to know exactly what to say, they lead fascinating lives, they have few if any problems. In contrast we feel unfashionable, inarticulate, and generally inept. The longer we stay, the worse we feel about ourselves and the more self-conscious we become.

The mistake we make at such times is comparing our "insides" to other people's "outsides." When we make these comparisons, we almost always judge ourselves unfairly. We draw conclusions based on surface appearances and mannerisms that probably don't accurately reflect reality. Just because people seem to have it all together doesn't necessarily mean they're more successful at living their lives than we are.

As we work on our self-esteem and it gradually improves, we become less vulnerable to our imaginations and the psychological traps they create from time to time. We realize that outside appearances are of small importance, while inner realities are all-important.

THOUGHT FOR TODAY: Don't compare your insides to other people's outsides.

How often we look upon God as our last and feeblest resource! We go to Him because we have nowhere else to go. And then we learn that the storms of life have driven us, not upon the rocks, but into the desired haven.

—George Macdonald

Change is unsettling, no matter what form it takes. We are bound to become upset by the breakup of a relationship, for example. But we can also become disconcerted by changes we welcome, such as getting married, or moving from a crowded apartment into a spacious home of our own. In either case we're likely to be thrown off-balance and, for a time, even to feel a sense of aloneness.

When we are overwhelmed by change, we can turn to God, the source of stability and serenity within us. By doing so, it is far easier to make whatever adjustments or adaptations are necessary.

Through our conscious contact with God, we can regain our equilibrium and become centered once again. If we rely on God and have faith in the rightness of His plan for us, the changes we face will take on new clarity and purpose.

When we turn to God, our sense of aloneness is lifted. He is with us, leading the way, providing the strength and courage to meet any challenges we may face.

THOUGHT FOR TODAY: In a life filled with change, God is my constant.

October 7

To listen well is as powerful a means of influence as to talk well.

—Chinese proverb

We've reached a point in our spiritual development where it has become second nature to want to help others. It's not always clear how to go about this, especially when direct opportunities aren't readily apparent. Yet there is a way to be of service every day: We can listen patiently and caringly to others.

Once we develop our listening skills and put them into action, we find that being attentive is one of the kindest things we can do for another person. Even when it's inappropriate to offer advice or provide solutions, our willingness to listen can be a most helpful and meaningful service. By listening carefully to someone, we demonstrate that we're genuinely interested in their problems, concerns, and joys.

Needless to say, nobody benefits more than we do by our willingness to listen. When we're open-minded and receptive to the feelings and experiences of others, we put ourselves in a position to learn from them. Perhaps most important, listening to others takes us out of ourselves and moves us along the path of spiritual growth.

THOUGHT FOR TODAY: The more attentively we listen to others, the less separated and different we're likely to feel.

Hatred does not cease by hatred, but only by love; this is the eternal rule.

—Buddha

Soon after I embarked on my spiritual journey, I became involved in a bitter legal dispute. During the proceedings I became enraged at my adversary. My immediate inclination was to lash out, as I always had in the past. But I dared not, for I knew the emotional price would be one I could ill afford.

Instead I worked hard at applying solutions I recently had begun to learn. I tried to "let go and let God," to practice forgiveness, and to release the person with love. But time passed and my resentment continued to torment me.

I turned in desperation to a knowledgeable friend. She suggested that I add a new dimension to my spiritual efforts by actually *praying* for the person. On several occasions my friend had asked God to provide "health, happiness, and prosperity" to those she resented. Additionally, she told me, in each case she imagined the person surrounded by an aura of "pure white light."

For several weeks I followed the advice. To my amazement and relief, my resentment was lifted. Today when I must pray for an adversary, it works no less effectively than it did the first time. What happens, I believe, is that my prayers "transport" the person from the realm of my resentful thoughts back to the realm of the Spirit, as one of God's children.

THOUGHT FOR TODAY: Prayer, especially for another, can free us of the bonds of resentment.

October 9

Let us not go over the old ground; let us rather prepare for what is to come.

—Cicero

You woke up this morning with an emotional hangover. You did something really unwise last night, and now you hate yourself for it. If only there were some way to go back in time and undo the damage.

But you can't go back, and regrets and self-punishment will only make it worse. The best thing to do is to put yesterday behind you by doing whatever you can to remedy the situation, by making amends if that's appropriate, by learning what you can from your mistakes, and by forgiving yourself.

Today is a new day, a chance for a new beginning. It is another golden opportunity to let go of the past, to put aside unrealized expectations, to forget about yesterday's disappointments. You can be open to new ideas. You can be free to concentrate on the present. You can become renewed—mentally, emotionally, and spiritually.

It is never too late in the day to begin. You can begin anew at any hour, wherever you are. At work, at home, or even on the road, at noon or at midnight, you can start again.

THOUGHT FOR TODAY: Today is another golden opportunity for a new beginning.

Pain is no evil. Unless it conquers us.

—Charles Kingsley

No one needs to be reminded that pain is an inevitable part of life. Whether it comes to us through trauma, loss, or as a result of our own behavior, we can't escape pain no matter how hard we try.

By reviewing our progress in life, it's easy to see that we have usually grown through pain. Some people, in fact, believe that pain is the "touchstone of growth."

Looking back, we may also realize how frequently we have caused our own pain, or compounded it by our thoughts, attitudes, and actions. We can remind ourselves, too, that emotional pain doesn't last forever—it *will* go away.

It's important to remember that we don't have to go through pain alone, nor do we have to rely only on ourselves in dealing with it. Certainly God will be at our side. We also can be helped by the suggestions and support of people who have had similar experiences.

Pain has the capability to either strengthen or destroy us, depending on how we respond to it. Often, the most effective response is acceptance. When we are able to accept our condition, we may be able to alleviate pain by removing the undeserved power we have given it.

THOUGHT FOR TODAY: Don't give pain the power to destroy you.

October 11

They have only stepped back in order to leap farther.
> —Michel Eyquem de Montaigne

We began our spiritual journey with the preconception that failure, at least as we understood it, was "bad." Over time we came to realize that many of our so-called failures weren't what they appeared to be, but in fact were necessary stepping-stones along the pathway of spiritual growth.

In the past when we willfully set self-seeking goals and failed to achieve them, we either continued to stubbornly pursue them, or eventually turned away in frustration and even rage. Today, in contrast, when we are not successful in achieving a certain objective, we are willing to consider the possibility that it was not meant to be.

Perhaps, for example, we have set a particular career goal. Despite our best efforts, the goal remains out of reach. These days, rather than feeling sorry for ourselves, we're more likely to accept the seeming failure as part of God's overall plan for us.

We have come to believe, through actual experience, that what God has in store for us will be far more beneficial than anything we could devise or even imagine on our own. That is why we continue to earnestly pray for His guidance, trusting that He will take us on to better things.

THOUGHT FOR TODAY: Within the context of God's plan, today's seeming failure may be a stepping-stone.

The selfish man suffers more from his selfishness than he from whom that selfishness withholds some important benefit.
—Ralph Waldo Emerson

It doesn't take a lot of insight these days to see how my self-centered actions and attitudes injured other people. Thoughtlessly, I rode roughshod over anyone who got in my way—from casual acquaintances at work to those I loved the most.

But I've also come to realize that my self-centeredness seriously affected the way I treated myself. I demanded a lot from others, to be sure, but I unreasonably and often mercilessly "took" from myself as well.

By standing in my own light, I constantly robbed myself of opportunity. Day after day and year after year, I treated myself harshly and with disdain, instead of being kind and patient. Driving myself relentlessly, I depleted myself in all areas. Whatever small degree of self-respect I once had was eroded by my self-seeking actions.

For the most part, providentially, that type of behavior has changed dramatically. I try to behave thoughtfully and generously not only toward others, but also toward myself. I pay close attention to my physical, emotional, and spiritual needs, taking actions that are enriching rather than detrimental.

THOUGHT FOR TODAY: Self-centeredness leaves no beneficiaries, only victims.

October 13

Time will bring healing.

—Euripides

When I once commented to a friend how well she looked, she smiled enigmatically but remained silent. I asked her what she was thinking about, and she replied that my compliment was a sharp reminder of what her life used to be like. "I was an escape artist," she explained. "I spent half of my time in doctors' offices and the other half in hospitals. You name it, I had it."

Illness, injury, and hypochondria were the ways by which she literally defected from the world when she couldn't deal with a specific situation or when she simply couldn't cope. She thought that the problem was her alcoholic husband. But as she learned later, the real problem was her reaction to his behavior.

The turning point came during a long-awaited skiing trip. Her husband careened drunkenly down the slopes—and she ended up with a broken leg because of her hysterical preoccupation with his behavior.

"I was in the hospital with my leg in traction and suddenly I understood what some people had been telling me for years. 'You're powerless over him and his disease,' they had been saying over and over. 'Release him—with love.'

"Thank God, that's what I was eventually able to do. My ex-husband hasn't gotten well yet, but at least I have. I haven't been in a hospital in years. The rest of it is out of my hands."

THOUGHT FOR TODAY: You are powerless over others, but not over the way you react to them.

Seize from every moment its unique novelty, and do not prepare your joys.

—André Gide

Special moments come our way when we least expect them. In fact, many of our most joyful experiences and exciting opportunities come as real surprises. We know intellectually that this is what often happens in life; yet despite our knowledge, some of us still try to manage and control the outcome of every event.

We have preconceived ideas about what we think "needs" to happen—and that's the way we approach most activities. The problem is we're so busy looking for, hoping for, and trying to influence future results, that we miss out on the uniqueness of the present moment and the possibility of surprise.

Let's say we've invited some friends to a party. Instead of relaxing and enjoying their company, as well as the fruits of our preparation, we worry and fret like mother hens over trivial details. Needless to say, this type of involvement can turn a potentially positive experience into a real chore.

The next time we find ourselves getting caught up in "management and control procedures," let's step back and allow things to happen the way they're supposed to.

THOUGHT FOR TODAY: Allow each moment to unfold in its own, sometimes surprising way.

October 15

Losing an illusion makes you wiser than finding a truth.
—Ludwig Börne

It was made quite clear to me, at the beginning of my recovery, that honesty in all areas was essential. It was vital to be aboveboard with the people who were helping me, but this principle had to be practiced unwaveringly in all other relationships as well. I was also told that the only way I could continue to recover and grow spiritually was to be rigorously *self*-honest.

Years later, I am still greatly challenged by this goal. I usually know almost immediately when I'm being dishonest with others, but it's much more difficult to become aware that I'm deceiving myself. In fact, the deeper I dig, the more unconscious self-deception I uncover.

Only after several years of recovery, for example, did I become aware that my motives for "people-pleasing" had to do with the desire for personal gain. More recently, I realized that my tendency to set unattainable work goals for myself is based on a need to feel important.

The more I discover, the more amazed I am by the elaborate rationalizations with which I sometimes justify my actions and attitudes. But I try not to be hard on myself as more is gradually revealed and I gain new insights. For I now believe that the pathway to self-honesty is an unending one.

THOUGHT FOR TODAY: Rigorous self-honesty is essential to recovery and spiritual growth.

Today I felt pass over me
A breath of wind from the wings of madness.
> —Charles Baudelaire

The day starts out okay, but by midmorning everything begins to unravel. Confusion and fear quickly take over. Soon you feel you can't cope for another minute. Panic-stricken, you wonder if you are having a nervous breakdown.

What's going on? It could, of course, be a number of things, or a combination of several—and it certainly can happen to anyone. Perhaps you're reacting to a major buildup of pressure at home and at work. You might be going through the belated backlash of a recent trauma. Or your sudden inability to cope could have been exacerbated by physiological considerations.

What should you do? First, don't keep it to yourself. As soon as possible, talk to someone you trust. This will help remove some of the fear and power from what you're experiencing.

Next, give yourself unrestricted permission to do whatever is necessary to make it through this difficult time. Put your physical and emotional well-being ahead of all other responsibilities and considerations. But by all means don't be hard on yourself for needing to do so.

You may not feel close to God. Try to remember, however, that your efforts to ask for His care and protection will be heard.

THOUGHT FOR TODAY: You need not go through anything alone—ever. Understanding and help are always close at hand.

October 17

The best mirror is an old friend.

—English proverb

Today we are blessed with very special friendships. We are free to be our true selves as we grow and work together. We have mutual trust and want the best for each other.

When we are on the verge of making a decision, and if we are uncertain, it has become second nature to check with our friends and seek their advice.

Since they care deeply about us, they don't hesitate to let us know when we're emotionally off the beam, or when the new scheme we've cooked up is pure fantasy.

The reverse is also true. Our friends are able to see, when we sometimes cannot, the progress we're making and the positive changes taking place in our lives. They are generous with their praise when they tell us how they feel about our growth.

Many of us have difficulty seeing ourselves as we really are, but we know we can usually see ourselves clearly through the eyes of trusted friends. It's a relief to be able to turn to them for comfort and reassurance. It's even more rewarding when we can be there for them.

THOUGHT FOR TODAY: If you would only be praised by true friends, you miss half their caring.

In actual life every great enterprise begins with and takes its first forward step in faith.

—August Wilhelm von Schlegel

Even after I had become willing to at least *try* to live by spiritual principles, it was difficult for me to understand what they were and how to apply them. I asked many questions, and was patiently given answers. But for months I simply couldn't put it together. What was being suggested to me was confusing to the point of incomprehensibility. It was as if I was being asked to believe that two plus two equals five.

Virtually every idea I was offered was contrary to what I had believed all my life. Almost every action that was suggested was the opposite of what I was used to.

For example, I expressed deep concern about my relationship with my family, about my finances, and about my shaky career. I expected to receive specific advice. But instead, I was told to work on my relationship with my Higher Power. When I complained bitterly about the way I was being treated by a relative, I expected sympathy. When it was suggested that I try to see how my character defects had contributed to the problem, I was baffled.

Slowly but steadily, it all began to make sense. Those spiritual tools began to work for me—but only when I stopped questioning how they could possibly be effective, and became willing to actually apply them.

THOUGHT FOR TODAY: Spiritual tools work when we are willing to work them.

October 19

A very popular error—having the courage of one's convictions. Rather it is a matter of having the courage for an attack on one's convictions.

—Nietzsche

As the world changes around us, we tend to change with it, particularly where dangers are concerned. We learn to take precautions when street crime increases. When we have to drive our cars during stormy weather, we don't need reminders to be careful. When science tells us certain substances are harmful, we avoid them.

Now that our outlook has become more positive overall, we see that certain attitudes are just as threatening to our emotional well-being as other hazards are to us physically. One such attitude is closed-mindedness.

When we are closed-minded, we resist change even when it is urgently required. We are likely to approach all problems with the same old ineffective "solutions." Beyond that, closed-minded people are often fearful, intolerant, and generally pessimistic.

Open-mindedness, in contrast, permits us to welcome change and to be receptive to new ideas and approaches. Open-minded people are better able to expand themselves mentally and spiritually. They are usually positive and easygoing. Because open-minded people become emotionally healthier and happier, they are more apt to help others and thereby better serve God and themselves.

THOUGHT FOR TODAY: Closed-mindedness enshrines ideas that are old, unworkable, and often damaging.

'Tis by no means the least of life's rules: To let things alone.
— Baltasar Gracián

"If it works, don't fix it." This widely used slogan is most commonly related to the procedures and machines in our lives—recipes, cars, copiers, and so on. Certainly no one can argue its validity in that regard. But the concept can also be valuable when applied, in a more personal way, to everyday living situations.

In the past, our tendency to question, analyze, and intellectualize things—often to the point of obsession—hobbled us in many areas. We were forever trying to fix and control people and situations, often in matters that had nothing to do with us. As a result, we frequently held ourselves back from fully experiencing freedom, serenity, and spirituality.

Why were we like that? The most probable reason is that our obsessive overinvolvement was born of egocentricity, and lack of trust. We've now discovered that one of the quickest ways to ruin a good thing is to arbitrarily and needlessly search out "flaws that need fixing."

As we've worked to become less self-centered—and more trusting of others, ourselves, and God—we've learned to do our best and then leave things alone.

THOUGHT FOR TODAY: If things are going well, let them be.

October 21

The greatest good you can do for another is not just to share your riches, but to reveal to him his own.

—Benjamin Disraeli

It has been a slow process. Only gradually have I become rid of much of my self-centeredness. The rewards of this new way of life have been myriad. Most of the changes concern the way I perceive myself, how I relate to others, and my ability to be comfortable and relatively free from fear.

One reward that remains unsurpassed is being able to get outside of myself by reaching out to someone still imprisoned by the same bonds from which I have been freed. I have found that the most effective way for me to help someone else is the simplest way—to share my *own* experience, strength, and hope.

Once, I remember, a man in early recovery revealed to me a litany of past wrongs. He was deeply ashamed and filled with self-loathing. He felt that he was "beyond hope"—that it would be impossible for him ever to progress from his below-ground emotional state.

I was able to let him know encouragingly, and empathetically, that I once felt exactly the same. I was able to help him see his "riches" by telling him what had been told to me: It's important to see and accept your faults, and to take responsibility for them, yes—but it's just as important to uncover and accept your assets.

THOUGHT FOR TODAY: Share your experience, strength, and hope to benefit yourself as well as others.

The desire of perfection is the worst disease that ever afflicted the human mind.

—Louis de Fontanes

Why do we so often pressure ourselves to perform perfectly in many areas—to be perfect mothers, fathers, sons, daughters, lovers; to have perfect bodies; to accomplish every undertaking with perfection?

Unfortunately, many of us have been taught to seek perfection, so we've gotten into the habit of expecting it from ourselves. Sometimes we feel that people will like us better if we're "perfect." Sometimes we simply don't realize what we're doing. And some of us subconsciously punish ourselves in our quest for perfection—by repeatedly setting the stage for failure.

In any case, when we strive to be perfect the results are predictable. Since complete perfection is impossible, we always fall short. Because we're so often dissatisfied with our accomplishments, we limit the opportunities to feel good about ourselves. Eventually we get caught up on a treadmill that prevents us from enjoying our jobs, our relationships, and life in general.

Clearly, the pursuit of perfection causes frustration and pain. These symptoms are completely reversible, however, if we give ourselves a break by simply trying to do our best instead of attempting to do the impossible.

THOUGHT FOR TODAY: Practice doesn't make perfect—it doesn't even make "perfect practice."

October 23

People are lonely because they build walls instead of bridges.
— Joseph F. Newton

We used to feel sorry for ourselves because we were so lonely. We now realize that our behavior served to purposely distance us from others, and we were therefore largely responsible for our own alienation.

Some of us kept people away by putting on airs of superiority. We pretended to be superintelligent; we were arrogant and overbearing experts on any and all subjects. We may have enforced our isolation by giving the impression that we were in total control of every detail of our lives. We didn't need anyone's help, we didn't need anyone's advice. We didn't need anyone, period. Sometimes we drove people away by behavior that was frightening or repugnant.

Whether we did these things knowingly or were unaware of our behavior, the underlying motive was the same. We had negative perceptions of ourselves, and were afraid that others would feel the same way if they got to know us.

Thankfully, we have found ways to raise our self-esteem, and no longer need to build walls around ourselves. We are now able to welcome others into our lives and are successfully putting loneliness behind us.

THOUGHT FOR TODAY: Ask yourself from time to time, "Am I unknowingly keeping others from getting close?"

The nicest thing about the future is that it comes one day at a time.

—Anonymous

Every one of us has goals and aspirations. We might long for that special person to become a part of our life. Or we've set our sights on a certain career objective. Perhaps we dream of financial prosperity. We may feel that we are ready for all of this right now, but let's remember, things really do happen when they are supposed to.

We're often told that everything occurs in God's time. We've found that this isn't just an abstract spiritual concept, but something that is taking place in our lives every day. God has a plan for each of us. His plan might well include exactly what we want for ourselves —or gifts that are beyond our imagination.

Whatever God has in mind isn't going to come to pass until we are ready for it. In fact, that's part of His plan. One day at a time, He is preparing us for what's to come in the future.

Day by day, God puts before us new experiences, lessons, opportunities, and challenges. That's His way, we believe, of preparing us for His future gifts. And only He knows when we will be ready to receive them.

THOUGHT FOR TODAY: What we are experiencing today is preparing us for what will happen in the future.

October 25

It makes a great difference in the force of a sentence whether a man be behind it or no.

—Ralph Waldo Emerson

Maintaining healthy relationships is one of our greatest challenges. That's why it's so important to periodically tune up or even overhaul our communication skills. One common cause of breakdown is the practice of sending out mixed messages—saying one thing, but meaning or implying something else.

Typically, our partner or spouse asks, "Do you mind if I go out tonight?" We reply by saying, "No, go ahead," but our intonation or body language conveys something quite different. We may utter a deep sigh and pause dramatically before we answer. Perhaps we have a pained expression on our face. Or we slam a drawer shut while we're responding.

Although mixed messages don't necessarily destroy relationships, they certainly don't do anything to enhance them. To the contrary, when we play this devious little game, it's usually because we want to be manipulative or controlling. We may try to make the other person feel guilty, sorry for us, or unsure of themselves.

If we find we are sending mixed messages, it's important to realize how unfair we are being by tap-dancing around the truth. If we want to keep our relationships healthy and growing, we have to strive for open and honest communications—in all situations, at all costs.

THOUGHT FOR TODAY: Mixed messages are manipulative.

It is with disease of the mind, as with those of the body; we are half dead before we understand our disorder, and half cured when we do.

—Charles Caleb Colton

Soon after I began my recovery from alcoholism, I was flooded with feelings of guilt and remorse for things I had done while practicing my addiction. I felt deep and genuine regret for my behavior and the harm it had caused. In addition, I was almost obsessively determined to "make up" for my past wrongs to others—for lost time, lost opportunities, and lost affection.

No less painful was my self-indulgent conviction that I had been so bad for so long that I would never be able to redeem myself.

One night that all changed for me. I heard another recovering alcoholic describe feelings that were identical to my own. Those feelings almost drove him back to the bottle, he said. "I realized just in time," he emphasized, "that the things I did while drinking were symptoms of my disease. I had to decide once and for all whether my alcoholism is, in fact, a treatable disease—or an unforgivable sin."

I have long since stopped punishing myself for having a disease, regardless of old ideas or outside pressures that briefly surface from time to time. I do what is right and good because it is right and good—not out of guilt or a need to make up for past wrongs.

THOUGHT FOR TODAY: I am not a bad person getting good, but a sick person getting well.

October 27

What shadows we are, and what shadows we pursue!
—Edmund Burke

A man I know was once walking along an empty beach, thinking about a "deal" he had just completed. He was filled first with self-confidence and then self-doubt; his mind shuttled back and forth between fantasies of enormous future wealth and fears of total failure.

Suddenly he stopped and looked around. He gazed toward the empty horizon and was awed by the ocean's immensity. He stared up at the clouds and was filled with wonder at their ever-changing grandeur. He looked across at enormous sand dunes formed of countless tiny grains; on distant bluffs he saw trees that had been shaped by the wind.

"I was taken aback," he recalls. "I felt a great sense of calm. For the first time in a long time, my sense of self-importance seemed to diminish, along with many of my expectations and fears.

"On that very special day," he adds, "I realized that although each of us is important in his own way, we sometimes have to look at the greater picture to see our own existence in true perspective. That's what I try to do as often as I can these days, and it really works for me."

THOUGHT FOR TODAY: Put it into perspective.

The highest wisdom is continual cheerfulness; such a state, like the region above the moon, is always clear and serene.
—Michel Eyquem de Montaigne

My intention today is to stay positive, trying not to let anything interfere with that important goal. If something unforeseen drags my spirits down, or if a boring task erodes my good humor, I'll remind myself that it's easier to approach and overcome these types of challenges with positive rather than negative energy.

If I'm forced to deal with a mean-spirited and abusive person—or if I'm placed in an unacceptable situation—I'm far more likely to maintain a positive attitude when God is on my mind. Time and again, experience has shown me that He will protect and care for me. Therefore, when I turn to Him, I can't help but be optimistic.

My intention today, moreover, is to share my positive energy with others, to be buoyant and lighthearted. If I am, I'll be better able to respond to those around me with warmth, kindness, and good cheer. Laughter will come easily. Hopefully, my optimism and high spirits will be contagious and I'll be good company to others. If I remain in a positive frame of mind, I'll certainly be good company to myself.

THOUGHT FOR TODAY: I'm far more likely to have a positive attitude when God is on my mind.

October 29

The time is always right to do what is right.
                              —Martin Luther King, Jr.

At times, in everyday situations as well as more serious ones, each of us is tempted to put off what we know must be done. Maybe we're afraid of the way people will react, so rather than risk confrontation or commotion, we look the other way. Or perhaps we hesitate to do what's right because we're uncertain of the results. In other instances, we may be unwilling to face the consequences because we know *exactly* what to expect.

No matter what fear-motivated excuse for delay we may have, it's always important to promptly take actions that reflect our hard-won values and principles. No one can accomplish this with perfection, of course, but we should be willing to do our very best. For as soon as we compromise or delay necessary action, our values begin to lose priority. If we continue our inaction, they may eventually become meaningless.

We do what is right for our own sake as well as the sake of others. When we adhere consistently to our values, we feel good about ourselves and are able to gain self-respect. But when we delay taking proper action because "the time is not right," the reverse is true and our self-esteem is undermined.

THOUGHT FOR TODAY: By doing what's right without delay, you feel right about yourself.

Freedom to live one's life with the window of the soul open to new thoughts, new ideas, new aspirations.

—Harold Ickes

Now that we've found solid footing in the world, we're less restrained in our approach to life. We're not afraid to steadily learn more about ourselves; we have a clearer awareness of what we want and where we are going.

God is a constant source of strength and good in our lives. We feel safe in the knowledge that He will guide us and care for us, no matter what. Because of our trust in Him and our growing self-confidence, we are free to do things that previously were impossible.

We are free and able to take risks—to explore our capabilities and inner resources—to have opinions and be assertive. Many of us have discovered hidden talents and have found the courage to pursue new careers.

We also have developed the honesty and self-awareness to challenge our limiting beliefs and ideas; our growing sense of security gives us the freedom to do so. We're no longer afraid to make mistakes, for we are willing to learn from them and to continue changing. We have the ability and desire today to pursue spiritual objectives that can never be achieved absolutely—patience, tolerance, understanding, and unconditional love.

THOUGHT FOR TODAY: Our trust in God frees us to do things that previously were impossible.

October 31

We lie loudest when we lie to ourselves.

—Eric Hoffer

It seems so easy to get away with lying. Perhaps that's why so many of us got into the habit and found it so hard to break. Sometimes we weren't even aware that we were lying. Our lies were disguised—as cover-ups, denial, rationalizations, or exaggerations.

We lied to avoid responsibilities and confrontations, to call attention to ourselves and gain approval, to smooth things over and make life simpler. Some of us reached the point where truth lost its meaning and lying became a reflex.

Since honesty with others and ourselves is so crucial in our lives today, what are some things we can do to stop lying and stay stopped? The first step is to acknowledge how harmful lying is to us, no matter what form it takes. We can then try to become aware of the ways in which we depart from the truth, and ask ourselves what we expected to accomplish in each case.

Some of us are able to break the lying habit by taking more direct action. When we find ourselves in the middle of a lie, we stop, admit what we are doing, and apologize. This can be embarrassing, to be sure, but it forces us to think twice before we tell the next one.

THOUGHT FOR TODAY: By their nature, lies are harmful to us, no matter how "necessary" or seemingly well-disguised.

Every man takes the limits of his own field of vision for the limits of the world.

—Arthur Schopenhauer

Few of us were ever actually jailed during our lives, yet we have endured another form of bondage. The bars of our prisons were constructed of selfishness, self-centeredness, and egocentricity. The locks were fashioned of closed-mindedness.

As long as we relied solely on such limited resources as self-will and determination—the conviction that we could manage and control our own lives—we remained imprisoned.

We were able to find freedom only when we focused less on ourselves and shifted our field of vision toward wider realms. We were able to gradually accomplish this by listening to the experience and advice of others—by asking God for direction and strength—and by making an effort to be of service.

As a result of these actions we found not only a way out, but a new way of life offering happiness, joy, and freedom beyond measure. It has been proven among us that so long as we continue to take certain simple actions, we can remain free of the bondage of self.

THOUGHT FOR TODAY: Action is the key to unlocking a closed mind.

November 2

To ease another's heartache is to forget one's own.
—Abraham Lincoln

In recovery we have made energetic and thorough efforts to rebuild our lives. Today we are joyous and serene most of the time, where before we were anxious and fearful.

Yet occasionally each of us is assailed by intense emotional pain. We do what we have been taught to do, redoubling our efforts to seek conscious contact with God, and taking action to help ourselves where we can. We try to be patient as we wait for God to bring guidance and comfort. But time passes and our pain increases. It seems that we've reached the end of our rope.

At such times we find the one thing that can bring immediate relief is reaching out to help a newly recovering person. Needless to say, it's not always easy to become even willing to do this. When we're absorbed in our own pain, the last thing we usually want is to get involved in someone else's suffering.

Yet if we are willing to make the initial phone call or volunteer the first reassuring word, such actions *will* change the way we feel. Almost miraculously we transcend our own pain and are able to gain a wholly new perspective. By moving outside of ourselves and into service, we are borne into a new state of consciousness.

THOUGHT FOR TODAY: When helping others, we often tell them exactly what *we* need to hear.

Experience is not what happens to a man. It is what a man does with what happens to him.

—Aldous Huxley

I'm learning that I don't have to react in the same old predictable ways when negative things happen in my life. I'm not a laboratory animal—I don't have to tremble at the sound of a raised voice or salivate at the tinkle of a familiar bell. Today I do have choices.

When I go through a bad experience, I can react as I always have, with self-pity. Or I can make the better choice of trying to learn from the experience, incorporating the knowledge into my future life and actions. That way, the trauma can be lessened—and my reaction tempered—if a similar event takes place again. It's even possible that my new knowledge can help me prevent such events from reoccurring. When I make the right choice, it's amazing how much I can learn—and the ways in which I can benefit—from experiences that on the surface are seemingly adverse.

Of course, all this is easier said than done. But it can be done if I remain self-aware and teachable. I find that I'm best able to handle adversity when I'm willing to change, when I try to accept life as it unfolds, and when I seek solutions rather than burying myself in the problem.

THOUGHT FOR TODAY: We gain humility by seeking and doing God's will to the best of our ability.

November 4

Procrastination is the art of keeping up with yesterday.
—Dan Marquis

From time to time each of us is guilty of procrastination. As we well know, it can manifest itself in many ways. Regardless of the extent to which procrastination affects us, we shouldn't take it too lightly.

What happens when we put things off? Nobody needs to be reminded of the sometimes deadly consequences of procrastinating in matters of health. But what's the harm in being neglectful or simply lazy in more routine and seemingly mundane matters?

Let's assume, in this vein, that your car has developed engine trouble. You're concerned but you don't want to be bothered. So you drive to and from work in the slow lane, with your fingers crossed. You keep procrastinating, and the longer you use the car the more loudly it knocks. Each day it gets worse, and your stress increases.

Finally, then, the inevitable happens—the car breaks down and you have to have it towed. It ends up costing several times as much in aggravation and dollars as it would have if you had handled it when you first noticed the problem.

The point is, of course, that every time we procrastinate it ends up affecting our lives negatively. When we put things off, in seemingly insignificant areas as well as important ones, we invariably pay the price.

THOUGHT FOR TODAY: There's always a price to pay for procrastination.

"Underneath are the everlasting arms." What child of God was ever permitted to fall lower than God's "underneath"?
—H. Gill

Some of us grow up with the idea that God is to be feared. As a result, we find it difficult to avail ourselves of God's power when we reach a point of surrender in our lives and admit our own powerlessness. If He is punishing and unforgiving, as we've believed, how can He help us? Why would He even want to?

In my own case, when I reached that point, it became necessary to reexamine and then begin to change my concept of a Higher Power. In the process I was offered several suggestions that helped me considerably.

Since I was free to develop my own concept—God as *I* understand Him—why not choose a loving, caring God? That's the whole idea, I was reminded.

I was also helped by remembrance of an "Irish Prayer," a blessing with this last line: "And may God hold you in the hollow of His hand."

Over a period of time that image has become very meaningful. It is poetic and memorable, to be sure; more importantly to me, however, it mirrors the reality of a loving Higher Power and His works in my new life.

THOUGHT FOR TODAY: God did not bring you this far so that He could drop you.

November 6

Hate the sin and love the sinner.

—Mahatma Gandhi

When we are wronged, we have a tendency to automatically characterize the person who has wronged us as mean, or bad. When we do this, there is a great deal of negative fallout, especially if the person is someone with whom we've been close.

The relationship is likely to suffer. And it soon becomes uncomfortable to be around the person, particularly in a work situation. Beyond all of that, when we "hate the sinner," we lose an important opportunity to practice understanding and forgiveness.

Certainly, it's difficult to avoid a hostile reaction when we've been wronged. It's even more difficult to turn a negative scenario—one that invites epithets—into a positive growth experience. But it is possible, and it's worth attempting.

First, we should consider the possibility that the person who wronged us was emotionally or spiritually off balance. Second, we should try to avoid retaliation or argument—otherwise we destroy our chance of being helpful. Finally, we should ask God to help us show that person the same tolerance, compassion, and empathy that we would gladly give to a physically sick friend.

THOUGHT FOR TODAY: It is in pardoning that we are pardoned.

The search for happiness is one of the chief sources of unhappiness.
—Eric Hoffer

At least once, we all have asked: "Why can't I be happy?" Perhaps we have felt, as many do, that it's possible to be happy all of the time—that there is a "bluebird of happiness."

It seems sad that some people spend so much of their lives trying to achieve the impossible goal of "living happily ever after." Even more unfortunate is that such people, driven by their fantasies, inevitably become even more unhappy as the result of this frustrating pursuit.

I also became discouraged when I perceived happiness as something you either have in its entirety or not at all. When I was able to seriously examine my beliefs and misconceptions, I realized that happiness comes during moments in a day, not as a "forever" thing.

I began to savor the individual moments and was surprised at how many there actually were: the satisfaction following a job well done; the sense of deep mutual understanding with a friend; the beauty of a sunset.

Today these moments of happiness come quite frequently. I am grateful that I can now recognize and appreciate them as the gifts they are.

THOUGHT FOR TODAY: Happiness comes a moment at a time.

November 8

Faith is the assurance of things hoped for, the conviction of things not seen.

—Hebrews 11:1

Sometimes we used to wonder about the substance of faith. We may have asked ourselves how it works, and what powers faith to answer prayer. Now that we have seen faith bring about previously impossible transformations in our lives and the lives of those around us, we no longer concern ourselves with such questions. Our speculations have become irrelevant. What is important is that faith *works*, and we know that from our own experience.

A man I know describes what happened to him. His addiction to alcohol was so acute that he had been able to sober up only when institutionalized or forcibly restrained. Yet one day he found himself getting through withdrawal while he was free, and while alcohol was available. "I found faith on my second day sober," he recalls. "I realized something was happening that was impossible without the help of God. It was clear that a Power greater than myself was keeping me from drinking."

Our faith can bring forth miracle after miracle. No matter how small or faltering we think it may be, our faith is a mighty spiritual force within us. Just as we press a button and expect electricity to flow into our homes, so we can open the channel of faith and expect God's infinite power to bring results in our lives.

THOUGHT FOR TODAY: Faith by its nature is mysterious. We need only know that it works.

The wrongdoer is often the person who has left something undone, rather than the person who has done something.
—Marcus Aurelius

We still shudder at the memory of those emotional hangovers. Anxiety was our constant companion, surrounding us like heavy fog. We often had the feeling that we would run aground. The problem was a buildup of unresolved issues between ourselves and others. We carried around an ever-weightier burden of bad feelings and lingering troubles.

The solution has turned out to be surprisingly simple. We've learned to take the time—each day—to honestly and forthrightly look at ourselves and to review unfinished personal business. We regularly ask ourselves if we've been unkind, prideful, or selfish in any way. We check to see if we have to make amends to anyone, if we need to clear up a misunderstanding or right a wrong. If the answer to any of these questions is yes, we map out a plan to promptly and thoroughly clean the slate.

It has gotten easier and easier to apologize, to admit and remedy mistakes, and to regularly inventory our character assets and liabilities. And now that we've found a way to prevent these unresolved issues from building up in harmful ways, we have far more peace of mind.

THOUGHT FOR TODAY: You can't afford the price of excess emotional baggage.

November 10

If error is corrected whenever it is recognized as such, the path of error is the path of truth.

—Hans Reichenbach

Once we get into the habit of taking daily personal inventory and promptly handling our unfinished business, we find our progress accelerates. This is how we learn and grow—by continually looking at ourselves to see where work is needed.

If, for example, we find that it is frequently necessary to apologize to someone or to correct the same mistake, it doesn't take long for us to get the message. Similarly, if we find a particular character defect is repeatedly causing us difficulty, we soon recognize and accept the necessity to change our behavior.

Through our daily inventories, we can also develop a solid and practical awareness of what works or doesn't work in our lives. We are then able to apply this knowledge in situations and interactions as they occur.

In other words, if we feel that we're about to "fall apart," we can take a few minutes to quiet our emotions. Or if we sense we're on the verge of doing or saying something unkind, we can stop ourselves before harm is actually done. If we've already gone too far, we are more willing to promptly admit and correct our wrongs.

THOUGHT FOR TODAY: Avoid emotional hangovers by taking a daily personal inventory.

Nature goes her way, and all that to us seems an exception is really according to order.

—Goethe

Whatever responsibilities I have today—whatever decisions I must make, whatever the demands on me—I will try to be conscious of God's divine timing and order.

If I become impatient while waiting for an outcome or response, I'll try to remember that everything in God's world happens when it is supposed to. I'll remind myself that the events of the day will unfold in His time, not mine, and that His plan and schedule is for the greatest good.

I may become momentarily overwhelmed by unexpected happenings that need my attention. I'll remember, though, that I am prepared and capable. God has confidence in me and never gives me more than I can handle.

What a comfort to know that His wisdom is guiding and regulating my day. What a relief to be aware that *I* don't have to solve all problems and meet all challenges through my own limited resources. I can turn to God.

Today I'm going to acknowledge God's loving presence and intelligence in all my thoughts and actions. I will keep in the forefront of my consciousness this reality: In all matters, great or small, God is in charge.

THOUGHT FOR TODAY: Everything in God's world happens how and when it is supposed to.

November 12

One self-approving hour whole years outweigh.

—Alexander Pope

"It was like I had a love-hate relationship with myself," a friend once told me, describing his past life. "At certain times I was totally egocentric—I felt and acted like I was the most brilliant, talented, and attractive person around. But most of the time I loathed myself. I thought I was the scum of the earth."

His egocentricity and attitude of superiority usually surfaced when he was with other people, my friend recalled. "Looking back, the whole idea was to get approval," he said. "But instead, my obnoxious behavior distanced me from them. When I was alone, that's when the other sick extreme took over—I couldn't stand myself."

My friend reached the point where he could no longer bear the painful consequences of his erratic feelings about himself. It was only then that he could take steps to bring about change.

"I had to work on both extremes, the egocentricity as well as the self-hate," he said. "In effect I had to wipe the slate clean and start over.

"I can't say that I have feelings of self-love yet," he added, "but I'm making progress. Right now it's kind of like a slow and gentle courtship, if you know what I mean."

THOUGHT FOR TODAY: Open your heart and mind to a new sense of wholeness and equality.

Fear is a slinking cat I find beneath the lilacs of my mind.
—Sophie Tunnell

It comes as a surprise to many of us that we don't know how to handle good fortune. When unusual opportunities or prosperity comes our way, we find ourselves reacting inappropriately. Instead of being excited and happy, we feel upset.

Fear is often the culprit when we have such unexpected feelings. We're afraid we won't be able to "live up to" our good fortune. We're afraid it will vanish as quickly as it came, and we're apprehensive about the changes that might be in store for us. Our most troubling and irrational fear, however, is that somehow a huge mistake has been made. We feel, deep down, that we don't deserve our windfall.

For some of us, clearly, good fortune can be as difficult to accept as adversity. But that doesn't mean we can't turn things around if we give ourselves a chance.

First, we can try to put our inappropriate feelings on hold. That way we can better see them for what they are—self-centered fear, rooted in old ideas. Instead of reacting quickly and self-destructively, we can take time to learn to accept our good fortune. Then, rather than focusing on our imagined unworthiness, we can try to become grateful for our bonanza and see it for the gift it is.

THOUGHT FOR TODAY: You deserve whatever good comes your way today.

November 14

God enters by a private door into every individual.
                                        —Ralph Waldo Emerson

A recovering alcoholic once described for me his frustration in trying to help a friend with a severe drinking problem. The young man first asked for help when he was attending college; he still owned a car and lived in a nice apartment. Based on his own recovery experience, my friend advised him that it would be impossible to stop drinking by willpower alone—that he must have spiritual help.

Although the young man tried to follow this advice, he returned to the bottle many times. Each time he lost something more and eventually he landed on the streets.

"I felt terrible for him," my friend recalled. "But it was beyond me why he couldn't get the message, why he had to sink so low."

At that moment I realized what is meant by the phrase, "It takes what it takes." Each of us reaches bottom—the point at which we surrender completely—in our own way and our own time. For some the bottom may be bankruptcy or a jail cell; for others, like my friend, it may be one too many humiliating moments. The process seems to have little to do with willpower, intelligence, background, or tolerance for pain—and everything to do with God's will and our readiness to accept Him in our lives.

THOUGHT FOR TODAY: It takes what it takes.

The love we give away is only the love we keep.
—Elbert G. Hubbard

When I finally decided to deal with my problems instead of running away from them, help was immediately available. I was amazed at the way others responded to my pain and reached out with empathetic suggestions. Especially surprising was the way people shared memories of their own suffering, taking the time to explain how and why things had gotten better.

To be honest, at first I was suspicious. I wondered what was in it for them and kept expecting to be asked for something in return. I simply couldn't understand why they seemed to *care* so much.

Not long afterward I found myself being helpful to a person suffering through the same problem that had seemed unendurable to me only a month earlier. It wasn't anything I had planned to do; it just happened that way. But it was a turning point for me.

I heard myself saying things that I needed to hear once again. By sharing my own experience and newfound strength—limited as it was—I reaffirmed for myself how far I had already come.

On that day I realized exactly why we care and reach out to each other. I saw clearly that it is by giving it away that we get to keep it.

THOUGHT FOR TODAY: Give to receive.

November 16

There is no witness so terrible—no accuser so powerful—as conscience which dwells within us.

—Sophocles

Guilt is like the toxic dust that lingers in the atmosphere following a volcanic eruption. Long after we have erupted in thought or deed, this powerful and poisonous emotion can block out the sunshine of happiness.

Sometimes we're haunted by guilt for months and even years. The act itself has long since been forgotten by everyone else concerned, yet we're still guilt-ridden. It doesn't seem fair. After all, we've done everything we can think of to make up for our reprehensible behavior.

We've made apologies and amends, face-to-face wherever possible. We've made financial restitution, if that's been called for. We've followed the advice of others and looked for patterns in our thinking and behavior that might have led to the deeds, and we haven't done anything even remotely comparable since. So why do we still feel guilty?

Perhaps it's because we haven't asked God's forgiveness and, no less important, haven't forgiven ourselves.

THOUGHT FOR TODAY: Self-forgiveness can help free us of guilt.

Trials are medicines which our gracious and wise Physician prescribes, because we need them; and He proportions the frequency and weight of them to what the case requires. Let us trust His skill and thank Him for His prescription.

—John Newton

For many of us, faith in a Higher Power came quickly in our new lives; it took only willingness on our part. Trust, on the other hand, developed more slowly, requiring not only an openness of heart and mind, but also experience born of action.

In our early recovery we weren't yet able to trust God's "prescriptions." We sometimes questioned the things that happened to us and the challenges that were put in front of us. "We've already been through hell," we complained. "What's going on? Doesn't He know how fragile we are?"

Now our trust has grown stronger, for we've come to realize that God never gives us more than we can handle. Experience has taught us that the adversities as well as the uplifting events in our lives take place neither a moment too soon nor a moment too late. They occur at exactly the right time and, thanks to a loving God, in our best long-term interest.

THOUGHT FOR TODAY: God never gives us more than we can handle.

November 18

In managing human affairs there is no better rule than self-restraint.

—Lao-tse

Life is filled with provocations, aggravations, and difficult people. We try not to get upset by them. We've learned time and again that when we permit ourselves to respond hastily or unrestrainedly, we're the ones who suffer—often greatly so.

But we're human and sometimes we can't help reacting angrily. At such times we may be tempted to lose our temper, lash out, or do something irrational.

There is something that could serve as a safety valve the next time you're on the verge of "losing it." Say to yourself, "Hold everything," and then take the time to think about what that means.

Just because someone else is making a fool of himself or herself doesn't mean you have to sink to the same level. So the first thing to hold is your tongue. If you remain silent there will be nothing to regret or feel guilty about later, but as we all know, it's hard to take back an angry outburst.

"Hold everything" also means to hold your temper. It's helpful to think of temper as a temporary onslaught of insanity during which we revert to our old ways. In fact, the next time you see someone lose his temper, watch closely to remind yourself just how damaging and foolish this type of behavior can be.

THOUGHT FOR TODAY: When you "hold everything," you can avoid "losing it."

Our most important thoughts are those which contradict emotions.
—Paul Valéry

It's easy to get swept away by negative emotions. When we're under the influence of such feelings, it always seems that things are much worse than they really are. And of course we're also unable to approach our problems rationally.

Sometimes even minor adversity can trigger a chain reaction. In a typical scenario, you are off to a very important appointment and the car won't start. The first reaction is panic. That leads to anger. From there you're likely to slip into self-pity, then into negative projection with its attendant fear, and ultimately to the despairing question each of us has asked at one time or another: "What's the use?"

We've all been there, but we don't have to go back if we don't want to. When that first negative feeling starts sucking us into the whirlpool of irrationality, there are several things we can try to do. First, we can move into the solution by turning to our intellect and away from our emotions. We can ground ourselves by bringing another person into the situation; even a phone call can be helpful in returning us to objectivity.

Another way to free ourselves is to make a list of options that can possibly solve the problem. Finally, we can remind ourselves that we have lived through far worse situations—that they've turned out fine, and this will, too.

THOUGHT FOR TODAY: The best first step is the one that takes us out of the problem and into the solution.

November 20

As in the physical world, so in the spiritual world, pain does not "last forever."

—Katherine Mansfield

I discovered early that no matter how badly I feel, I won't go on feeling that way forever. This realization has become an important principle in my life—a useful tool that can be applied to many circumstances and situations.

During previous attempts at giving up my addictions, I was always abruptly confronted by my unbuffered feelings. The emotional pain was amplified by the pangs of withdrawal, and before long I was forced back into my seemingly protective cocoon.

I finally reached the point where I conceded to myself that the addiction was no longer an alternative—I knew, deep down, that it would never "work" again. In a short while I again began to experience fear, anxiety, loneliness, and depression—those same feelings that always had pushed me over the edge. But this time, probably because I had admitted defeat, I discovered that the feelings only *seemed* unbearable. I was able to hang on, and the pain passed.

These days when I go through rough times—difficulties at work, for example, or even grief—I know that if I do what is in front of me the painful feelings will pass and serenity will return.

THOUGHT FOR TODAY: This too shall pass.

Our plans miscarry because they have no aim. When a man does not know what harbor he is making for, no wind is the right wind.

—Seneca

Lately we've been disappointed with ourselves. We've been haunted by a sense of impending failure, to the extent that we're beginning to dread facing the days ahead. We're taking less pleasure in many of the things we've been doing at home and at work.

Could it be that we have developed unrealistic expectations of ourselves? Are we setting standards and making demands on ourselves that are impossible to achieve? Or perhaps we're taking on too many responsibilities, without first thinking them through.

When we set unattainable goals, we automatically position ourselves to fail and become discouraged. When we push beyond our limits, we cheat ourselves out of the chance to feel good about our accomplishments— because there's no time to acknowledge them. There's no time, either, to learn from our mistakes; we're too busy getting involved in the next project.

If we want to get back to enjoying our activities, we have to stop putting so much pressure on ourselves. By recognizing and accepting our limitations, we can better deal with the demands over which we have less control. And we'll be able to function more efficiently at whatever we do.

THOUGHT FOR TODAY: Don't expect yourself to do any better than your best.

November 22

Relationships are like crucibles, in which our character defects rise to the surface.

—Anonymous

When we finally decide to do something about our discomfort, most of us have only limited self-perception. We're not really sure why we're uncomfortable. All we know is that we often mistreat others, especially those we love—and we rarely feel good about ourselves. We also tend to think of our unacceptable behavior in extremes; generally we see ourselves as "bad" people who need and want to get "good."

As we grow less confused, we become aware that the solution to our problems has nothing to do with going from bad to good. We learn that we have an array of character defects—anger, envy, and greed, to name some—that are frequently triggered by self-centered fear. It's a great relief to us when we're taught that one by one these defects can be acknowledged, identified, and worked on. We can "name them, claim them, and dump them."

Our character defects always have revealed themselves most clearly in our relationships with others. As our recovery progresses, we are able to work on these flaws with ever greater effectiveness. Today, it is in our relationships that we can see the greatest positive change in ourselves.

THOUGHT FOR TODAY: Character flaws need not be permanent, but can be "named, claimed, and dumped."

The worship most acceptable to God comes from a thankful and cheerful heart.

—Plutarch

Thanksgiving week is special for us in many ways. Because of God's grace, we are able to be reunited with our families and friends. It is with a deep sense of gratitude that we gather together in celebration. We know that our warm thoughts and caring behavior toward one another are a true reflection of God's love.

As we participate in the events of the month, we each take time in our own special way to thank God for the blessings He has so freely bestowed. In offering thanksgiving, we're filled with a growing awareness of the abundance in our lives. As we express gratitude for each gift, others come flooding to mind. We are elevated in consciousness, so that we recognize and rediscover His numerous blessings within and around us.

We are grateful that we have been brought together safely. We are grateful for our mutual love and understanding ways. We are grateful for our individual and collective successes. But most of all we are grateful for God's presence—not only during the holiday season, but through all the days of our lives.

THOUGHT FOR TODAY: Remember the true meaning of Thanksgiving.

November 24

He that will not apply new remedies must expect new evils; for time is the great innovator.

—Francis Bacon

It's pleasurable and relatively easy for me to give advice to other people. Because I've been through similar problems and situations, I often know just how they feel and can offer solutions that have worked for me. I also try to give credit where it is deserved: When I see that people are being helped because of my advice, I'm often grateful to God that I can be a channel for His grace.

But when new problems surface in my own life, or when old obsessions and attitudes haunt me, it's sometimes difficult to put the principles I've learned into action. In other words, I don't always practice what I preach.

Sometimes, for example, I wait until my back is against the wall or I'm in great pain before I surrender and ask for God's help.

Why do I wait so long? One reason, probably, is that I tend to deny I'm in pain or actually facing a real problem. Sometimes I decide it's not that serious and will work itself out. Or, most likely, I get so involved in the problem I forget about seeking a solution.

Despite my lapses, the fact is that I don't remain in pain anywhere nearly as long as I used to. So even though it's bad once in a while, it's still a lot better than it's ever been.

THOUGHT FOR TODAY: Live in the solution, not the problem.

I dread success. . . . I like a state of continual becoming, with a goal in front and not behind.

—George Bernard Shaw

When people have reached certain enviable goals, we often say that they "have arrived." We assume that life will be a breeze for them—that they've got it made. We feel that we too will have arrived when we achieve one or more highly desirable goals: when we get married, have a baby, get promoted to a senior position, stop drinking, lose thirty pounds, move to the country, and so on.

Although it's admirable and perhaps vital to work for such goals, the idea that any of us can ever "arrive" is a fallacy. It requires discipline, responsibility, and hard work to care for a baby, contribute to a marriage, maintain a weight loss, or "stay stopped" from drinking. And just because we achieve these objectives, it doesn't mean life will be problem-free or that we'll even be happy.

Moreover, recovering people have special needs. Many illnesses can't be cured, but can only be arrested a day at a time.

None of us—whether we are recovering or simply trying to improve our lives—can ever achieve absolute success. Better than that, we can achieve multitudes of successes, one following the other a day at a time.

THOUGHT FOR TODAY: Thank God for this successful day.

November 26

When we are tired we are attacked by ideas we conquered long ago.
          —Nietzsche

Many things that influence the way I think and feel are beyond my control. However, I do have control over my basic health needs. I find that the choices I make in this area dramatically influence the quality of my emotional sobriety.

I wasn't always aware there are choices. I was convinced, for example, that the only way to control my weight was to go all day without eating. I'd indulge myself with the fix of an angry outburst because I "needed to let off steam." I'd isolate myself for days believing that being alone enhanced my creativity. I'd allow myself to become overtired to the point of distortion. As a result, during early recovery I experienced frequent mood swings, lapsing into the type of behavior I had come to abhor.

I talked to other recovering people about my problem. They told me that when they let themselves get too *H*ungry, *A*ngry, *L*onely, or *T*ired (HALT, as they put it), they experienced the same mood swings and became vulnerable to the dangers of old ideas and actions. My immediate thought was, "How corny! *My* problems are deeper and need more sophisticated solutions."

But I was willing to experiment and before long saw how right my new friends were. Now, taking advantage of simple solutions like HALT, it's much easier to stay on the beam.

THOUGHT FOR TODAY: HALT: Don't get too *H*ungry, *A*ngry, *L*onely, or *T*ired.

We can easily forgive a child who is afraid of the dark; the real tragedy of life is when adults are afraid of the light.
—Plato

We lived in ways that allowed us to escape reality. If our chemical or behavioral dependencies didn't enable us to actually avoid the real world, they buffered us by altering our consciousness of it. When we gave up our dependencies, we found that reality was even more baffling and frightening than before. We were unnerved and, for a time, became sorely tempted to fall back into our old ways.

What was it we were so afraid of? For one thing, we dreaded taking responsibility; we'd never been willing to do that before. Some of us also feared interacting with other people. Moreover, we didn't want to face what we had become. At that point we still were unwilling to accept things as they were.

Facing reality is one of the first major challenges of our new life. It comes on us very quickly. This is a critical time for us, because the decisions we make will assuredly affect the speed and ease of our future progress.

Clearly, the best choice is to face reality head-on. The initial tests of our willingness may well be the hardest, but by facing them courageously, we will gain strength and faith to continue doing so as a matter of course.

THOUGHT FOR TODAY: No matter what you do, reality is here to stay—and is meant to be enjoyed.

November 28

Prayer does not change God, but it changes him who prays.
— Sören Kierkegaard

Like so many people, I began my new life with a certain amount of skepticism toward the concept of a Power greater than myself. I expected to be chided by my newfound advisers, but to my surprise they nodded understandingly.

By admitting defeat and expressing willingness to be changed, they told me, I already had taken a major first step. Lovingly and with great patience, they guided me along a new pathway—not toward their God, or the God of my family, but to a God of my *own* understanding. For me, that guidance was the key to faith.

In all honesty, my first prayers were fumbling and rather hollow. I wasn't yet willing to turn my will and life over to God's care. But I continued listening to those who came before me. I simplified my prayers, beginning each day by asking God to be with me, and ending each day by thanking Him.

Gradually my belief and trust grew strong; I found God within me and could see His works in my life. Through my own experience I eventually understood what others had meant in my shaky early days when they told me, "I came, I came to, I came to believe."

THOUGHT FOR TODAY: Willingness is the key to acquiring faith in God as you understand Him.

Deliberate with caution, but act with decision; and yield with graciousness, or oppose with firmness.

—Charles Caleb Colton

Making decisions—for many of us, it's among the most difficult and even dreaded things we have to do. Yet it doesn't have to be that way, not if we're willing to take a close look at the way we ordinarily approach decision making.

If we're really honest about it, the first thing we'll realize is that making a decision isn't anywhere near as painful as *not* making one. Even when we're not quite certain in the case of a "close call," at least we take action when we decide. If we sit on the fence paralyzed by doubt, we don't go anywhere.

For some of us, the inability to make important decisions is the result of our unwillingness to take responsibility. And we often pay an added price for that—we're more easily influenced by others into taking actions that may not be right for us.

The ability to make decisions without undue anguish seems to improve in direct proportion to growing self-awareness and self-honesty—along with our willingness to take the steps necessary for change and progress. It also improves as we learn to trust ourselves and others. We are best able to confidently and comfortably make decisions when we learn to trust God, by listening to His guiding voice within us.

THOUGHT FOR TODAY: Making a decision isn't nearly as painful as *not* making one.

November 30

We must muster the insight and the courage to leave folly and face reality.

—Albert Schweitzer

Many otherwise sensible people cause themselves endless frustration by stubbornly adhering to their delusions and fantasies. Because they believe certain things ought to be true, they insist that they *are* true—even in the face of overpowering evidence to the contrary.

A typical case is the suffering alcoholic who has been arrested twice, three times, or more for drunk driving, yet as a symptom of the disease denies having a problem. Another example is the person who year after year pours money into a failing business—yet adamantly insists, even as the family's security is shattered, that "it's going to work."

It's sometimes hard to give up our cherished dreams, illusions, and fantasies. But we have to try to be honest with ourselves about such things, facing the fact that they can not only hurt us and those around us, but even lead to our destruction.

Once we become self-honest, it can then be helpful to seek guidance from someone we trust—preferably someone outside of the situation. Following that, we have to become willing to put aside our illusions and let them go once and for all. If something doesn't work, it doesn't work—be it drugs, a "perpetual motion machine," or a bad relationship. The more quickly we recognize it, accept it, and act on it, the better off we'll be.

THOUGHT FOR TODAY: To deny reality doesn't change reality.

334

Long years must pass before the truths we have made for ourselves become our very flesh.

—Paul Valéry

We realize that it's more important to approve of ourselves than to have the approval of others. Yet again and again, we become hurt and angry because we aren't getting enough approval from someone. It's one thing to know something intellectually, but it's quite another to respond to that knowledge at a deeper level. In fact, only when our "head knowledge" becomes "gut knowledge" are we able to consistently react with maturity.

If there were some quick and easy way to bring this about, we could avoid many inappropriate reactions, not to mention a lot of pain and frustration. But the reality is that this somewhat mysterious process is a gradual one. It requires a considerable amount of self-honesty, self-awareness—and patience.

In my own case, when I realize that I'm once again reacting immaturely and inappropriately, I try to "freeze frame" the moment and briefly step out of it. That way I'm able to see the situation—and my role in it—with greater clarity and objectivity. By doing this repeatedly, my intellectual knowledge slowly but steadily becomes a working part of my nature.

THOUGHT FOR TODAY: When intellectual knowledge becomes gut knowledge, we take a giant step toward maturity.

December 2

There are two kinds of people in the world: those who come into a room and say, "Here I am!" and those who come in and say, "Ah, there you are!"

—Anonymous

The best way to get something we want is to give that very same thing to someone else. That applies to love, forgiveness, understanding, hope, and kindness—as well as many other qualities. This principle for living is one of the most significant spiritual truths we have learned, and its origins can be traced far back in recorded history. One of the most inspiring and well-known prayers of all time expresses it this way:

Prayer of St. Francis of Assisi

Lord, make me an instrument of your peace.
Where there is hatred, let me sow love;
Where there is injury, pardon;
Where there is doubt, faith;
Where there is despair, hope;
Where there is darkness, light;
And where there is sadness, joy.
O Divine Master, grant that I may not so much seek
    to be consoled as to console;
To be understood as to understand;
To be loved as to love;
For it is in giving that we receive—
It is in pardoning that we are pardoned;
And it is in dying that we are born to eternal life.

THOUGHT FOR TODAY: Each time you reach out to another, you reach out to God.

We fear something before we hate it; a child who fears noises becomes a man who hates noise.

—Cyril Connolly

If it is true that we have undergone dramatic changes in attitude, why do we still react so negatively to some things? How is it that we can actually feel hatred in certain situations? When we honestly examine such feelings, we can see that the things we hate are often the ones we most fear.

Many of us have vivid memories, for example, of "holidays gone wrong"—sometimes to the point of disaster. Our fear of getting through the holidays remains so strong that we still wish we could avoid them entirely—we continue to "hate them." The same may be true of other situations that have been extremely unpleasant for us in the past—new social experiences, visits to doctors or dentists, and so on.

Since we must get on with our lives, what can we do in such cases to avoid discomfort in the future?

Understanding the nature of our fears can be an extremely helpful beginning. By honestly confronting our fears instead of allowing them to remain disguised as other, perhaps "more acceptable" feelings, we can learn to walk through them. And by so doing we can make it possible for our previously negative reactions to become positive ones.

THOUGHT FOR TODAY: Hatred is often fear's disguise.

December 4

The mind can not long act the role of the heart.
                              —Duc de La Rochefoucauld

Several years into my sobriety, I took on a writing assignment that required a long automobile commute several times a week. The work went extremely well and soon increased in volume. The company's chairman became concerned that the heavy driving was too much for me. He arranged to have the firm's helicopter pick me up close to my home. Instead of fighting traffic for several hours, I had only to drive ten minutes to the airstrip.

I was the only passenger in the giant Sikorsky that first morning and evening. As we soared above the crowded freeways, I could hardly believe my good fortune. Just several years earlier I had been a face-in-the-gutter drunk. "Look at me now!" I thought.

Months passed and the rides became almost routine. Then, one morning, "my chopper" was late. It was scheduled to pick me up at eight, and it was already five past. I looked at my watch repeatedly. I began to pace back and forth. There was no sign of the helicopter. It was eight-fifteen and I was getting really annoyed.

At that point I began to smile. Soon I was laughing out loud. How quickly we can forget, I realized. And how easy it can be to take God's blessings and miracles for granted.

THOUGHT FOR TODAY: Accept God's gifts graciously, and take no blessings for granted.

No man is an island, entire of itself; every man is a piece of the continent, a part of the main.

—John Donne

Today our close and caring friendships are bright spots in our lives. When we look around us, it's hard to believe how reluctant we once were to accept help from others. But at the time, because of our fears, we had little choice.

Some of us were taught to be totally self-sufficient; we grew up believing it was wrong to live any other way. We were afraid we'd appear weak or incapable if we didn't insist on handling everything ourselves. Others among us couldn't accept help because we felt unworthy. Deep down, we were convinced we didn't deserve the time and attention of others.

All of that began to change as we gradually became less prideful, and felt more deserving of good. We started opening up, and even took comfort in the idea that we are all connected to one another in important ways.

We realize today that while it is possible to live in isolation, we can't flourish as human beings unless we interact with others. In fact, much of the progress we've made up to this point is the result of being able to accept the help, experience, and strength of our fellows.

THOUGHT FOR TODAY: Accepting help is not a sign of weakness, but an opportunity to further our progress.

December 6

The world is God's epistle to mankind—His thoughts are flashing upon us from every direction.

—Plato

Sometimes we get so caught up in everyday routines and responsibilities that we lose sight of God's infinite power. We limit ourselves by devoting most of our time and energy to our jobs and possessions.

Of course, there's nothing wrong with doing the best we can at what we do, and feeling good about the things we have. But we shouldn't let these things become walls that shut out our view of the larger world, the world of the Spirit.

When we bring God into our activities, they can become much more meaningful and satisfying. We're frequently inspired and uplifted at work and in our relationships. We get more out of life because we approach it with a true sense of direction and inner calm.

When we live in the larger world we are more often aware of God's power and His willingness to bring about miracles in our lives. We recognize and are grateful for His works, instead of taking our blessings for granted or seeing them as the result of mere chance.

By recognizing that each day's accomplishments and successes are far more God's than our own, we appreciate these gifts in an entirely new way.

THOUGHT FOR TODAY: Today's blessings are not the result of chance, but the gifts of God.

And if your friend does evil to you, say to him, "I forgive you for what you did to me, but how can I forgive you for what you did to yourself?"

—Nietzsche

Throughout the years we've heard again and again that when we harm someone, we're really harming ourselves. Never have we been more aware of the truth of this maxim than we are today. Never have we been more willing to apply this principle in our lives.

The reason for this, thankfully, is that we've become highly sensitive to the consequences of our behavior. We've learned to count to ten before we act explosively or slide into a hostile state of mind. We've progressed to the point where we know exactly what happens to us when we're angry, unkind, or hurtful toward others. Because of this knowledge and experience, it's much easier to avoid behavior or attitudes that can cause us guilt, remorse, or pain.

Beyond that, we're simply no longer willing to pay the price for behavior that's harmful to others and ultimately to ourselves. This is what we mean when we say, "The road gets narrower."

Contrary to what some people may think, this is not a limiting way of life. Just the opposite is true. Now that we have solved many of our basic problems and dilemmas, we're able to move on to new spiritual levels. The result is that we are enjoying greater freedom and broader horizons than ever before in our lives.

THOUGHT FOR TODAY: The narrowing road leads us to greater freedom.

December 8

Love is an expression and assertion of self-esteem, a response to one's own values in the person of another.

—Ayn Rand

In spite of my occasional major outbursts, frequent lapses, and ever-present negative attitude during my former life, I tried to be a loving person. I see now that my ability to love others, and to receive love from others, was severely limited because of the way I felt about myself.

I was filled with self-hatred for so long that my emotions were usually awry. My character defects—such as impatience, intolerance, and anger—made it impossible for me to offer love unconditionally. Beyond that, I've come to realize, my motives were often not what they appeared to be: I sometimes acted lovingly toward family members so they would forgive me; I frequently acted lovingly toward friends, acquaintances, and even strangers in order to use them. At the same time I was unable to freely accept love from others because of my deep-down conviction that I was undeserving.

Today, because I try to follow spiritual principles and do what is right and good, I've been able for the most part to cast out self-hatred and replace it with self-love. As a result it is far easier for me to feel empathy and compassion for others, and to be kind and loving to them with no strings attached. I am also able to accept God's constant love as well as love from my fellows when it is offered.

THOUGHT FOR TODAY: Love must first be nurtured within before it can be freely given and received

The principal part of faith is patience.

—George Macdonald

There is no timetable for faith. We each come to believe at different times and for different reasons. As time goes by and our faith grows, we begin to apply it with increasing frequency in our lives.

In the past we were knowledgeable, and capable of intellectual realizations. We knew, for example, what it was like to become obsessed with something. We may even have realized that our obsessions were totally self-destructive.

When we acquire faith, we go beyond knowledge and realization. We discover a way to do something about our character flaws. We learn that when we've had enough of the pain, we can ask God to remove the flaw—and that He will do so if we're genuinely willing to give it up.

Because of the intensity of the pain, naturally we want immediate relief—after all, we are only human. At such times we have to remember just how faith works—patience on our part is a vital requirement.

It is true that God always *does* help. It is true that relief always *does* come. But it is also true that these manifestations of God's power take place in His time, not ours.

THOUGHT FOR TODAY: Patience is not a cross to bear, but an essential ingredient of faith.

December 10

The rung of a ladder was never meant to rest upon, but only to hold a man's foot long enough to put the other somewhat higher.

—Thomas Huxley

You're clean and sober now. You feel so much better, even though it's only been a short while. It's great to wake up with a clear head and remember exactly what you did the night before.

Now the holidays are fast approaching and you're beginning to get nervous. You've been invited to a company Christmas party. You want to go, but you're afraid.

You talk about your predicament with friends who have been sober longer than you. Your questions tumble out: "What if somebody notices I'm not drinking and asks why?" "What if my boss insists I have one with him?" "What if I'm tempted?"

Your friends are helpful and reassuring. They've been through it themselves, so they know exactly what to tell you. By the time you arrive at the Christmas party, you're well-prepared and considerably less fearful. You have club soda, and when someone asks why you're not drinking, you reply casually, "I've already had enough." Later you smile at your private joke.

The boss never does ask you to join him. And when you spot a few people who are falling-down drunk, you're grateful to be upright and have your wits about you. As you drive home you thank God for being at your side during the evening.

THOUGHT FOR TODAY: You don't have to drink, use, or indulge—no matter what.

I am not afraid of tomorrow, for I have seen yesterday and I love today.

—William Allen White

Our pasts are being transformed from seeming liabilities into valuable assets. This is coming about through strenuous efforts to clear away yesterday's wreckage and, in the process, to learn as much as possible from previous experiences.

We gain knowledge by completely and fearlessly reviewing our lives. We achieve deeper insights through open communication with others who are willing to share their experience and knowledge.

More and more is being revealed along the way. It has become glaringly obvious, for example, that our problems were caused largely by our own actions and attitudes. We can also easily see how our self-oriented behavior contributed to damaging and even destroying relationships in all areas. We have been able to uncover and identify the character defects that require work if our lives are to continue improving.

These are some of the awarenesses that help us to live comfortably today. By taking the lessons of the past—even our most recent past—and promptly applying them in practical ways to unfolding situations, we often are able to avoid repeating mistakes and to prevent situations from getting out of hand. Because of the past, we are able to enjoy the present and face the future with confidence.

THOUGHT FOR TODAY: The past can become one of your most valuable assets.

December 12

Each man can interpret another's experience only by his own.
—Henry David Thoreau

I always kept my fears and anxieties to myself. Sympathy wasn't what I wanted, for it only added to my feelings of apartness. As for empathy, I had no true idea of what it meant.

Most of all, I was afraid that others wouldn't understand and might even laugh at me. Consequently, I remained isolated and usually felt a deep sense of aloneness.

In the first few days of my recovery, I tentatively shared several painful fears with another person. It was then that I was offered the most reassuring phrase I've ever heard: *"I know."* I immediately felt warmer and more comfortable inside. For the first time I had the sense of being "a part of"; it was a turning point for me.

The more I disclosed of myself over time, the more empathy and understanding I received, and the more fellowship with others I gained. The time came when I, too, was able to offer comfort and reassurance by saying those two magic words—"I know."

These days when someone confides his or her secret fears or concerns, I feel most helpful when I can relate my own similar feelings or experiences. "I know"—those are the kindest and most empathetic words I can offer anyone.

THOUGHT FOR TODAY: It takes one to know one; it takes one to help one.

How calmly may we commit ourselves to the hand of Him who bears up in the world.

—Jean Paul Richter

There are days when it is easy to be upset by the surface wrongness of things, when life seems unfair and unjust. Those are the times when we can profit greatly by reminding ourselves to "wear the world as a loose garment." This means approaching the day with the conviction that God has a purpose for the world, and that all is fundamentally well.

When we wear the world as a loose garment, we are reassured by our deep and abiding trust in God. We are able to put aside our concerns and know that everything will work out for the best as long as we try to seek and do His will.

Once we grasp this concept in a broad sense, we can then learn to apply it in very practical ways. When we wear our relationships as loose garments, they are bound to improve in every area. At home and at work, we become less sensitive and uncompromising. It's far easier to accept other people as they are. When we focus on the belief that all is fundamentally well, we are not as likely to take every little thing personally or every eventuality too seriously.

THOUGHT FOR TODAY: Wear the world as a loose garment.

December 14

One must be a god to be able to tell success from failures without making a mistake.

—Anton Pavlovich Chekhov

In the past we saw only one side of failure. Failure meant falling short—performing ineffectively—being unsuccessful. Failure was always something to be ashamed of.

We've since discovered that failure as a personal concept has far more to do with individual *attitude* than it does with fixed rules. Whether or not we fail is determined by our specific objectives—and the way we approach them—rather than by an arbitrary set of standards inscribed on a wall somewhere.

Let's say that we set out to improve our relationship with someone. During what we had hoped would be a conciliatory discussion, we lose our temper and a heated argument erupts. After reviewing what has taken place, we see what role we had been playing all along to contribute to the problems in the relationship.

Whether or not we have failed in such situations depends on us and our motives. We haven't failed if we're sorry for our past behavior. We haven't failed if we have an honest desire to let God guide us to better ways. We haven't failed if we apply our new awarenesses and continue to try to improve the relationship.

THOUGHT FOR TODAY: As long as we're willing to learn from our so-called failures, we can be assured of successes.

Meet the first beginning; look to the budding mischief before it has time to ripen to maturity.

—William Shakespeare

In almost every area of our lives things were constantly getting out of hand. We thought we were doing just fine in our relationships at home and at work, but then suddenly we'd find ourselves at the center of a full-blown emotional upheaval. All too often our checks began to bounce. Out of the blue, a minor health problem turned into something major.

These crises almost always came as surprises. We'd ask ourselves, "How did this happen?"

Today we know exactly how they happened. We let things go, for one reason or another, until they finally exploded in our faces. Sometimes fear or procrastination kept us from taking constructive action. Most often, however, things got out of hand because we simply didn't see trouble coming.

Thankfully we don't live that way anymore. Through self-honesty and self-awareness, we've learned to quickly identify potential problems. Then we nip them in the bud before they have time to bloom. In relationships, for example, when we feel even slight tension we try to loosen things up through improved communication. We meet responsibilities squarely and try not to over-extend ourselves physically, emotionally, or financially.

THOUGHT FOR TODAY: It's far easier to take care of small problems than to find your way out of major crises.

December 16

The future enters into us, in order to transform itself in us, long before it happens.

—Rainer Maria Rilke

When people ask me how I stopped drinking, I usually go through a litany of dates, events, and institutions leading up to the day I asked for and received help. Invariably, I feel afterward as if I didn't really answer the question. That's because it is almost impossible to comprehend, let alone describe, what actually happened to me.

Although I had tried many times to stop drinking on my own, I inevitably failed. What occurred the last time, however, superseded my personal endeavors.

My perception today is that toward the end I had begun to concede my powerlessness over alcohol. I was close to surrender, and to a true willingness to change.

Yet the subsequent events had nothing at all to do with *my* resolve, actions, or willpower. They had everything to do with the power of God. He achieved for me what I had been unable to do for myself.

It's not for me to know, but this is what I believe happened following my surrender: God stepped in and relieved me of my obsession to drink—even though I denied His very existence. The actual events are irrelevant, since specifics cannot do justice to the miracle.

THOUGHT FOR TODAY: Surrender, not willpower, sets the stage for recovery.

The afternoon knows what the morning never suspected.
-Swedish proverb

We were able to admit complete defeat only when the quality of our lives reached an all-time low. Ironically, however, because things had gotten so bad, it also seemed impossible that they could ever improve. Our skepticism was compounded by the many desperate but unsuccessful attempts we previously had made at changing.

When we disclosed our fears, people acknowledged them with understanding. "We know just how you feel," they told us. "We've been there." And they advised us, in simple terms, "It's going to get better, and here's HOW: *H*onesty, *O*pen-mindedness, *W*illingness."

It turned out they were absolutely right. Gradually, but most definitely, things did change in all areas— because we were willing to work for the changes.

We have since found a new happiness, peace, and purpose. But the greatest joy of all is being able to offer encouragement to yet another person who is as filled with disbelief and apprehension as we once were. We are able to say, with sincerity, "It's going to get better," and from our own experience know that it is true.

THOUGHT FOR TODAY: HOW = *H*onesty, *O*pen-mindedness, *W*illingness.

December 18

We are always in the forge, or on the anvil; by trials God is shaping us for higher things.

—Henry Ward Beecher

"At times it was as if all my character defects had come to life," a friend told me. "The dark side of my personality took over. Everything seemed distorted, and I felt alienated and self-destructive."

Each time he suffered this experience, my friend tried to deny his feelings and rationalize his actions. Secrecy became all-important, even though he knew that we all have our dark sides. "I was afraid of the gorilla in me. Each time he came out, I tried to stuff him back in his cage before he did too much damage. God forbid anybody should see him."

"So what finally happened?" I asked.

"He'll always be a part of me," my friend said in all seriousness. "But now I feel differently about him. Things changed when I could finally confide in somebody at a deep and honest level. With the help of that person, I was able to really explore my destructive personality.

"I reached the point where I could face the gorilla," my friend added. "I eventually accepted him as part of myself and, as strange as it may sound, I even embraced him. When I did that, he lost his power."

THOUGHT FOR TODAY: The cage within me, where I stuff my painful feelings, can become the cage around me.

. . . That is what learning is. You suddenly understand something you've understood all your life, but in a new way.
—Doris Lessing

People in every culture are taught almost from infancy the difference between right and wrong. We learn that it is "right" to be honest, courteous, and kind—and that it is "wrong" to lie, steal, or be hurtful to others. As children, our primary motivation in acting rightly is the avoidance of punishment. Later on, we're generally motivated by conscience as well as the mores of society.

As we grow spiritually, our awarenesses expand and intensify. We see more clearly how our actions and occasional compromises affect our lives and the lives of others. Consequently, we understand right and wrong in an entirely new way.

Today when we practice right rather than wrong, our motives go far beyond a desire to avoid punishment or a guilty conscience. We practice honesty, patience, and tolerance, for example, because they work in our lives. *Dis*honesty, *im*patience, and *in*tolerance do not work—and never will.

Because of our new understanding and more highly developed motives, we do what is right in order to feel better about ourselves, to live comfortably, and because our spiritual growth depends on it.

THOUGHT FOR TODAY: Motives are as important as actions.

December 20

God is a circle whose center is everywhere, and its circumference nowhere.

—Empedocles

Today I will make every effort to be conscious of God's presence and to be grateful for His blessings. In my meditation I will try to be receptive of His will for me. In my prayers I will seek strength to carry it out.

Throughout the day I will remember that God is always near. I will seek His wisdom and guidance in all the decisions I make. I will try to meet all challenges by availing myself of His sustaining power.

When I am with others I will try to gratefully reflect God's presence by acting with kindness, patience, and understanding. By giving my love and offering my ideas in ways that can be beneficial, I will respond to His grace. I will affirm the fact that God's qualities prevail and can be freely exchanged among His children.

At day's end I will quiet all thoughts and cares and turn my entire attention to God. Through meditation, I will seek His continued guidance, and through prayer I will once again express my gratitude for His blessings.

THOUGHT FOR TODAY: God doesn't vacation; His guidance and strength are always available.

*By all means sometimes be alone; salute thyself; see what thy
soul doth wear; dare to look in thy chest, and tumble up and
down what thou findest there.*

—William Wordsworth

For years our lack of self-confidence cast deep shadows
over our lives. Whenever we set out to accomplish
something, a voice within insisted that we could not.
Because of the way we worked against ourselves, facing
life's challenges was so much harder than it needed to
be.

Although few of us have been able to resolve this
problem entirely, we continue to make steady improvement. We remind ourselves, often, that when we dep-
recate our capabilities or talents, we're perceiving
ourselves dishonestly.

The way to overcome our distorted views, we have
found, is to give ourselves credit for things we have
done well. Each day we acknowledge our accomplishments, no matter how small they seem. We make
conscious efforts to honestly assess ourselves.

Instead of automatically projecting failure, we prepare
ourselves for success. We do this by setting realistic goals,
and by following through with the actions necessary to
realize them. We build on the things we do best.

When we are offered encouragement, we try to believe it, accept it, and use it. We are learning to trust
our friends—and ourselves.

THOUGHT FOR TODAY: By honestly assessing our
capabilities and special skills, we can build self-confidence.

December 22

People become house-builders through building houses, harp players through playing the harp. We grow to be just by doing things which are just.

—Aristotle

How grateful we are to be free of the destructive behavior patterns that kept us in bondage most of our lives. We were impatient, angry, and unfair to others for so long that we believed such feelings and actions were unalterable parts of our personalities. Eventually we stopped expecting anything different from ourselves.

It came as a great relief to discover that the traits we had accepted with resignation were not necessarily permanent. To the contrary, we were offered specific ways to bring about dramatic changes in our relationships with others. Step by step we learned to identify our harmful behavior patterns, to acquire willingness to give them up, and to ask God's help in becoming free of them.

Just because we had gone that far didn't mean we could expect immediate and automatic changes, it was explained. Still more effort was required. True progress could be achieved only if we *acted* in faith, applying the principles we had learned situation by situation and person by person.

We became just by doing things that are just. We became fair, patient, and understanding by acting fairly, patiently, and understandingly.

THOUGHT FOR TODAY: Even the most miraculous changes manifest themselves a new day at a time.

The greatest of faults, I should say, is to be conscious of none.
—Thomas Carlyle

For actively addicted people, blaming others and past or present circumstances is a common form of rationalization and denial. As martyrs, we were guilt-givers. We almost always used other people as foils to practice our disease. The refrains are familiar: "If you had a childhood like mine . . ." "If you were married to someone like . . ." "If you went through what I went through . . ."

But self-styled martyrdom is not the exclusive province of those who are chemically or behaviorally dependent. Just about anybody can choose martyrdom. Anybody can avoid taking responsibility for his or her life by styling himself or herself as a victim of circumstance.

Apart from the actual suffering that martyrs impose on themselves, their attitudes and behavior invariably bleed into every relationship in their lives. Old relationships remain tainted, while each new one is bound to become tainted. This is because a large part of any prolonged interaction needs to be based on sympathy or even guilt for the martyr.

Of course, there is another way. In our new life we've learned to put aside blaming others, and to take responsibility for our own problems. By practicing forgiveness, understanding, and compassion for those we once blamed, we try to resolve our past and get on with the business of living.

THOUGHT FOR TODAY: The first step out of martyrdom is the step you take into the now.

December 24

Man is the only animal that laughs and weeps; for he is the only animal that is struck with the difference between what things are, and what they ought to be.

—William Hazlitt

Is my life successful? Before I can answer, it's necessary to define what I mean by success. Do I still measure progress by my salary, my possessions, my popularity? Or have I learned to measure success in terms of such spiritual goals as character building, tolerance, understanding, and service?

Am I still gauging my success, even in spiritual pursuits, by comparing my growth with that of others? Or have I realized that the journey for each of us is highly personal and individual—that we each had a different starting point and move forward in God's time.

So is my life successful? Even though I've defined my terms, the question is still unanswerable, for it implies life in its entirety. A more pertinent question is, am I successful today? This is what really matters, because any progress I make is achieved one day at a time.

Yes, my life is successful today because of my faith and trust in God, and my efforts to seek and do His will. My life is successful today because I am willing to continue pursuing spiritual objectives, even though my reach will always exceed my grasp.

THOUGHT FOR TODAY: My life is successful today, thanks to God.

As a countenance is made beautiful by the soul's shining through it, so the world is beautified by the shining through it of God.

—Friedrich Jacobi

Christmas has finally arrived. For weeks we have been celebrating the season and awaiting this very special day. There has been a great deal of planning and preparation, up until this very morning.

We have decided to approach Christmas Day with a sense of wonder and joy. We have had great expectations, but now we are going to put all of them aside in order to enjoy the day as it unfolds. Even if our circumstances are not exactly as we would have wished, we will focus on the spirit of the holiday.

The true spirit of Christmas, we have discovered, comes from deep within ourselves. It flows from our ability to exchange love and joy with others, rather than from what we unwrap, eat, or drink.

We're grateful that we're able to feel this way, that we don't have to dwell on expectations or wishes. For our joy today will come from a willingness to share our Christmas spirit with others, to reach beyond ourselves in whatever ways we can to help make today as special for others as it is for us.

THOUGHT FOR TODAY: The true spirit of Christmas comes from deep within ourselves, where we have found God.

December 26

We should give God the same place in our hearts that He holds in the universe.

—Cicero

Many people take comfort in anecdotes or parables that have special meaning to them. When they are burdened in some way, these stories help them regain perspective and remember their priorities. A friend of mine tells one such story . . .

She answers the doorbell in the morning and is greeted by a man dressed in a tuxedo and top hat. He leads her down the driveway toward a gleaming white limousine and helps her into the backseat. "Everything is perfect," my friend says. "All my needs are taken care of. I sit back and relax. Even though there's traffic and the road is a little bumpy, the ride is as smooth as can be."

But soon the traffic becomes aggravating. The ride gets bumpier as the limousine accelerates. "Now we're speeding, weaving between the other cars," my friend recalls. "Suddenly the limo careens off the road, straight toward the cliff. It goes halfway over and just teeters there above the ocean.

"I look around in panic," she adds, "and realize to my dismay that I had gotten into the driver's seat once again. Everything was fine while I was willing to let God do the driving. The minute I took control, that's when I lost control."

THOUGHT FOR TODAY: My path will be smooth and my journey peaceful if I look to God today.

Love does not dominate, it cultivates.

—Goethe

Now that we've come to depend more on God, we find we're far less dependent on others. And because our needs for emotional security are being met in the best way possible, self-seeking has begun to diminish. Consequently our relationships in all areas are greatly improved.

In the past our insecurity and self-seeking usually caused one of two things to occur. We were either too dependent upon people, or we insisted on dominating them.

Today we realize that if we expect too much from others, they will inevitably fail us. Unlike God, people are fallible—they simply can't meet our unending demands for security. Similarly, we now see that when we constantly try to control others, either by manipulation or outright domination, they are bound to rebel. In either case the aftermath for us is more insecurity, hurt feelings, and resentments.

When we are overly reliant on people, we sabotage the possibility of having satisfactory relationships. We've learned that real partnership can be achieved only when we try to determine what we can put into a relationship, instead of what we can take from it.

THOUGHT FOR TODAY: When your relationship with God is right, it is likely that all your relationships will improve.

December 28

If the only tool you have is a hammer, you tend to see every problem as a nail.

—Abraham Maslow

For many years prior to my recovery—in fact, for most of my life—I lacked tools for living. I dealt with just about everything on my terms, using guile, hostility, and dishonesty to get what I wanted. Because I had never learned to understand myself, I felt lost in the world. Because I didn't know how to express my feelings, or even to identify them, I often behaved in ways that further alienated me. The most painful lack was my inability to interact with others.

It's difficult to pinpoint exactly when I began learning how to live comfortably. However, at some point I gained enough humility to become teachable.

As I became willing to listen to others and to be honest with myself, I gradually acquired a set of tools for daily living. I learned that I was not at the center of the universe—I could begin to see myself in perspective. I found ways to become more self-aware, to come to terms with the past, to acknowledge and become free of my character defects. All of this became possible only when I made God a part of my life.

THOUGHT FOR TODAY: You have a spiritual tool kit to solve all the problems of living.

Fear is faithlessness.

—George Macdonald

When we first gave up our dependencies, we faced an array of painful new fears. Without our chemical or behavioral "armor," many of us had difficulty handling the simple responsibilities of everyday life. Because of these fears, our ability to function was often limited. We had to relearn, sober, basics that most people take for granted—such as making phone calls, handling banking transactions, or returning merchandise to stores.

Somewhat reluctantly, we shared our fears with newfound friends. They said that such difficulties were common in early recovery. Most of them had gone through similar fears; they promised that time and experience would bring improvement.

Then our friends urged that we try the simple and effective solution of replacing fear with faith. Whenever we were fearful, they explained, we could find courage and strength by remembering that we are not alone—that God is with us and we are surrounded by His care and protection.

As we put this principle into practice, our faith strengthened and deepened. Our fears diminished and eventually disappeared as we gradually gained self-confidence. Today we are more comfortable for the most part. But when new fears occasionally surface, we know just what to do.

THOUGHT FOR TODAY: Replace fear with faith.

December 30

Life has taught me to think, but thinking has not taught me to live.

—Aleksandr Ivanovich Herzen

We used to think about our problems endlessly. We'd decide to do something about our jobs, marriages, or various situations Then we'd sit down and *think.*

We'd start out by trying to organize our thoughts, and we might even make some progress. Invariably, though, our project would get out of hand. We'd search fruitlessly for causal connections. We'd go off on tangents, and soon we'd start thinking about unrelated matters. Eventually, if we kept it up, we'd get to the point where we couldn't *stop* ourselves from thinking. Our problems and dilemmas then became tormenting obsessions.

Thankfully, we've now learned to apply spiritual solutions to life's sometimes perplexing or troublesome situations. And along the way, we've been able to put our intellects and thought processes into perspective.

We realize that our minds are gifts, and that they have enormous capabilities for positive accomplishments. But we're also aware that they have limitations and, in fact, can sometimes exacerbate our problems. These days we try not to become overly reliant on our intellectual powers in the sense of "thinking" our way through life. Instead, we allow our thoughts and actions to be guided by our ever-deepening spiritual resources.

THOUGHT FOR TODAY: Think about spiritual solutions.

Real generosity toward the future consists in giving all to what is present.

—Albert Camus

It's the last day of the year and the eve of a new one. For most of us this means it's a time of reflection. It is also a time to review our progress—to face up to our shortcomings, but also to acknowledge our assets.

Throughout the holiday season many people overindulge in various ways. The most commonplace excess—and the least recognizable—is overindulgence in the idea that, starting at midnight tonight, *everything will change.*

We make lists of all the things we're going to do, stop doing, or do differently. We make fervent resolutions of the ways in which we'll improve ourselves. We have high hopes for the "new year."

Wanting to change is well and good; as we all know, it is essential if life is to be fully enjoyed. Whatever we do, though, we shouldn't forget that change is best undertaken one day at a time. In that spirit, it might be more productive to think tonight about January 1 rather than the entire year ahead.

Perhaps most important, we don't have to wait until the end of a year—or, for that matter, until the end of a day—to become willing to make a new beginning.

THOUGHT FOR TODAY: Happy New Day.

Index of Authors

367

368

369

Index of Subjects

About the Author

The author of A NEW DAY chooses to remain anonymous, a practice consistent with recovery program philosophy. He has written several successful books with a combined total of more than 1 million copies in print, including A DAY AT A TIME, a classic work in recovery literature.